Thomas Dunkenberger

Tibetan Healing Handbook

A Practical Manual for Diagnosing, Treating, and Healing
with Natural Tibetan Medicine

Translated by Christine M. Grimm

D0817797

LOTUS PRESS

SHANGRI-LA

Important Note: The information presented in this book has been carefully researched and passed on according to our best knowledge and conscience. However, the author and publisher assume no liability whatsoever for damages of any type that may occur as a result of the application or use of the statements in this book. The information in this book is intended for the education of those interested in this topic.

The author, **Thomas Dunkenberger**, is a healing practitioner. For the past fifteen years, he has worked with energetic medicine, the Eastern variety in particular. During this time, he has become familiar with Tibetan medicine in theory and practice during lengthy visits to Nepal and India. One of the ways he deepened his experiences has been through advanced studies at the Samyê Ling monastery under Professor Dr. Thubten Phuntsok, as well as with Dr. Barry Clark. Thomas Dunkenberger communicates with various Tibetan physicians and healers on a regular basis. He lives and practices medicine in the Allgaeu region of Germany.

First English Edition 2000
©by Lotus Press
Box 325, Twin Lakes, WI 53181, USA
The Shangri-La Series is published in cooperation
with Schneelöwe Verlagsberatung, Federal Republic of Germany
©1999 by Windpferd Verlagsgesellschaft mbH, Aitrang, Germany
All rights reserved
Translated by Christine M. Grimm
German editing: Sylvia Luetjohann
Cover design by Kuhn Graphik, Digitales Design, Zürich, Switzerland
Interior illustrations by Peter Ehrhardt. On page 3 by Kuhn Graphik, Digitales Design, Zürich, Switzerland

ISBN 0-914955-66-7
Library of Congress Catalog Number 00-131115

Printed in USA

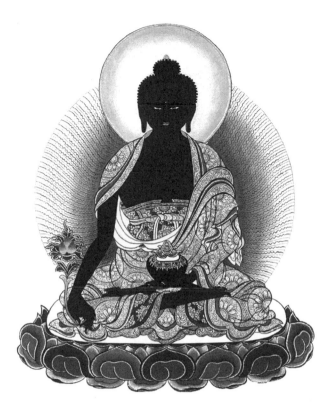

*May all sentient beings
be aware of the healing energy within them as a natural source of
strength that is freely available at any time*

DEDICATION

FOR MY BELOVED COMPANION
HEIDI MAYROCK

Table of Contents

Section IV
Diagnosis in Tibetan Medicine 145

Section V
Therapeutic Measures 173

Acknowledgments

I would like to express my deepest thanks to Dr. Trogawa Rinpoche for his spiritual accompaniment. Without his beneficent energy, this book would not have appeared in print. From the bottom of my heart, I would like to thank my teacher and friend Dr. Barry Clark for his helpful explanations. He understands how to communicate Tibetan medicine in a lively, humorous, and open manner.

I would also like to thank the Tara Rokpa Institute at the Samye Ling Monastery, as well as Professor Thubten Phuntsok, who teaches there, for their helpful explanations. Moreover, I sincerely thank Dr. Nel de Jong (Amsterdam), a physician for Tibetan medicine, and Professor Dr. Pasang Yonten Arya (Milan) for their assistance.

Butter

*Butter can be made from milk
because it contains the necessary fat.
We cannot make butter from water.
The golddigger finds the gold in the rock and not in the wood.
In the same way, striving to be like Buddha is only meaningful
because the Buddha-nature already exists in every living being.
If this potential did not exist,
all attempts in this direction
would be a waste of time.*

JAMGÖN KONGTRUL

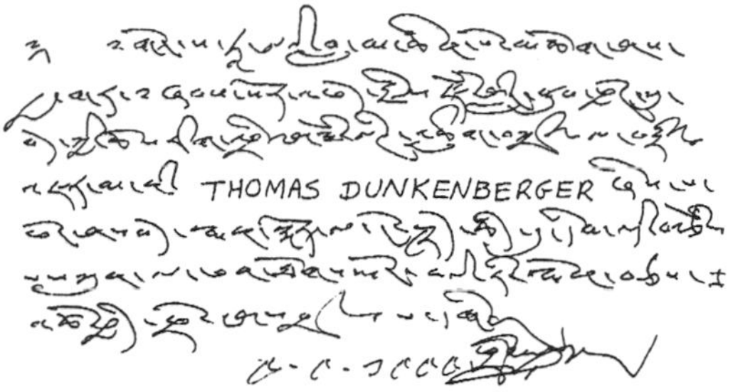

[handwritten Tibetan text]

THOMAS DUNKENBERGER

Preface

"Since the arrival of His Holiness the Dalai Lama in India, a solid bridge and connection between the Tibetan religion and culture and the Western world has been established.

This has created the basis for the publication of this introductory book to Tibetan medicine by Thomas Dunkenberger.

May this book prove to be helpful and effective for the good of all. My hopes and prayers are directed toward this goal."

September 9, 1999
Dr. Trogawa Rinpoche
(DIRECTOR OF THE CHAKPORI TIBETAN MEDICAL INSTITUTES, DARJEELING/NORTHERN INDIA)

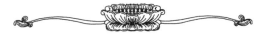

Foreword

– By Dr. Pasang Yonten Arya –

A new publication on Tibetan medicine is always welcome. I am particularly pleased about this current book by Thomas Dunkenberger because I am certain that it will prove to be distinctly helpful and valuable to those individuals in the West who would seriously like to study Tibetan medicine, as well as for the general reader. Thomas Dunkenberger has studied both Tibetan Buddhism and Tibetan medicine for many years under some of the most distinguished Tibetan lamas. In addition, he has translated several works on Tibetan medicine into the German language.

In ancient times, Tibetan medicine developed from the natural wisdom of the Tibetan people. However, the teachings of Gautama Buddha were responsible for the renewal of this knowledge and provided its ultimate form. The heart of Buddhist spirituality and the explanations of the laws and the nature of the psychophysical correlations imprinted these ancient medical teachings in terms of their ultimate orientation.

Tibetan Buddhism teaches that the mind controls and regulates the microorganism. The mind also furnishes the movement of the essential, meaning the central dynamic force, which leads to formation of the three energies *(nye pa)*.

In harmony with the three inherent psychological and emotional characters, this extends in a natural manner to the development of three "divisions" or dimensions. These energies (or humors) create and regulate both the psychophysical and the psycho-pathological complex and are called *rLung*, *mKhrispa*, and *Badkan (Péken)* in Tibetan medicine. These are usually called "wind," "bile," and "phlegm" in Western translations.

This book by Thomas Dunkenberger is certain to make a substantial contribution to the understanding of this venerable medical system.

June 24, 1999
Professor Dr. Pasang Yonten Arya Tendi Sherpa

(DIRECTOR OF THE NEW YUTHOK INSTITUTE OF TIBETAN MEDICINE, MILAN/ITALY AND FORMERLY PROFESSOR AND DIRECTOR OF THE MENTSEE-KHANG TIBETAN MEDICAL INSTITUTE, DHARAMSALA/INDIA)

How to Use This Book

Traditional Tibetan medicine represents a very extensive and distinctly complex system of naturopathic diagnosis and therapy forms. This book has the objective of introducing readers to this rich knowledge in an easily accessible and largely practice-oriented form. Consequently, it is not only aimed at individuals who provide treatment but also lay people interested in naturopathy. Moreover, it offers people in this latter group the opportunity to consider their own type of constitution with its respective strengths and weaknesses by carefully adjusting behavior and eating habits, for example.

To do this, I recommend that you fill out both of the questionnaires printed in the appendix of this book as an introduction to the topic. The first of these tests will help you determine your basic constitutional or bodily-energy type. The overview of the basic types: "Which Bodily Energy Type Best Describes You?" (see pg. 31ff. and 236f.) will prove to be quite illuminating for this purpose. If you have health complaints, the second test can help you determine where the imbalance is and which of the bodily energies may possibly be present to an excessive degree.

In the corresponding chapters, you can then read how to influence these disorders by sometimes amazingly simple means through behavior and eating habits. Easy-to-understand descriptions regarding the effect of the elements and seasons, as—well as the characterization of our most common foods according to the type of taste, medicinal effect, and special areas of application represent just a few of the possibilities that can make a decisive contribution to maintaining and/or restoring your own health. By largely dispensing with culturally specific characteristics and translating the information into Western terms (for example, an expanded selection of recommended foods), this book is very valuable in the practical sense. Even the methods and evaluation criteria of the pulse and urine diagnosis are explained in a way that is easy to grasp. This makes it possible for the readers to perform both of these themselves with some practice.

Tibetan medicine is closely interwoven with the Buddhist way of thinking. This has also been taken into consideration in the corresponding chapters so that readers interested in Buddhism will also learn new information. However, it is not at all necessary to be a Buddhist in order to gain much fundamental knowledge, as well as practical benefits, from this venerable but timeless store of knowledge.

Introduction

Because of the increasing public interest in the humanitarian and political fate of the Tibetan people, a magnificent jewel of Tibetan culture—"The Aquamarine Light of the Eight Branches of the Science of Healing" or in short: Tibetan medicine—has increasingly received the opportunity to shine in the West.

In this system of medicine, there are aspects of ancient Indian Ayurveda, traditional Chinese medicine, ancient Greek-Persian medicine, as well as the underlying Bon-Shamanism of ancient Tibet. Together with the spiritual values of the Buddhist culture, this has been woven into something completely new. Out of this synthesis, Tibetan medicine has assumed a comprehensive form of its own. For example, the form of urine analysis practiced here is only found in Tibetan medicine. The teaching on embryology uses a depiction of the fetus in the weekly steps of development, but this development is only described in monthly stages in the ancient Indian Ayurvedic depiction.

In addition, many moments of the depth psychology-energetic approach are integrated into this tradition in a way that has been "discovered" in the West only during the course of the 20th century and is unequaled to a certain degree. This form of healing science has served the Tibetan people in an excellent way for centuries. Tibet's physicians and remedies were known and continue to be known and praised far beyond its own borders.

We live in an age where increasingly more people, in the West as well, are recognizing their very own healing potential, which is inherent to every being. As a result, they are turning to a corresponding way of living and eating, as well as to the paths of naturopathy for support and optimization of this force. A truly holistic medicine like Tibetan naturopathy represents a great enrichment to this approach. The depiction of Tibetan medicine in this book is solely based on historic traditions. I have consciously refrained from adding any attributes of other healing systems that could possibly change the meaning. When these attributes are mentioned, I have clearly described them as such. Mixing various systems is only sensible when the foundation of each individual system is understood.

Although Tibetan medicine must certainly be comprehended within its own context, it is not necessary to become a Buddhist in order to benefit from it. Buddhism is a philosophy for perceiving our own potential and achieving all-encompassing compassion. This means that every type of dogmatism is foreign to the inner nature of Buddhism. However, the spiritual aspects of our reality and the diseases that we may possibly experience should never be neglected. As a truly holistic system, Tibetan medicine connects the mental and physical aspects into a whole and also offers the corresponding treatment methods.

Those who would like to learn Tibetan medicine usually first study the *Gyushi* (Tib. *rGyud bzi*). The four fundamental medical treatises or tantras are included in this title. The first tantra is called the Root Tantra. It offers a brief summary of the entire system of medicine. This is followed by the Explanatory Tantra, in which the same correlations are explained again in detailed form. The extensive Oral Instruction Tantra offers the most specific form of explaining the system and is completed with the fourth tantra, the Final Tantra. Among other things, this discusses the external therapeutic methods in a comprehensive manner.

Before the invasion by the Chinese and the flight of the Dalai Lama in the year 1959, there were an abundance of commentaries on the individual aspects of these tantras. However, only a relatively small portion of these texts still exist. The Tibetan tradition—namely, of memorizing all important texts—has largely contributed to the preservation of this valuable knowledge.

There is no doubt that Tibetan medicine represents a complex system, and so the question is repeatedly asked: "This is all so tremendously diverse and difficult. So where should I start reading and learning?"

This book gives you an introduction to the fundamental correlations and mentality of Tibetan medicine. The description is intended to offer the readers the opportunity of observing themselves within the scope of this medical system, determining possible imbalances in their energies, and drawing the appropriate conclusions with respect to the best way for them to eat and behave. This introductory book naturally does not claim to be a complete depiction of Tibetan medicine. Yet, if you comprehend and also apply the correlations, diagnosis procedures, etc., introduced here, you will have a good survey of the possibilities for optimizing your own bodily energies. Then you can turn to the literature that will further deepen your knowledge. The diagnostic procedures introduced in this book are all quite easy to apply. However, they should not entice us into making our own diagnosis. Instead, they are meant to help in achieving a deeper understanding about ourselves, as well as our modes of behavior, etc., and influencing how we live our lives in an appropriate manner. The two blossoms that develop from a conscious lifestyle are health and a long life. The three fruits that they produce are prosperity, contentment on the basis of wisdom, as well as spiritual development in a positive way.

A Brief Historical Survey

As frequently occurs with historical events, there are various approaches to the history of Tibetan medicine, depending on the respective point of view. The generally accepted version is that the historical Buddha Shakyamuni manifested as the Medicine Buddha (Tib. *Men-la*, Skrt. *Baishajya*). He held the medical teaching lectures in the form of a dialog between two emanations of himself—Rigpé Yeshe as the emanation of his heart (meaning the spiritual aspect), as well as Ji-lé-kye as the emanation of his speech—as tantric initiation.

Some sources claim that Kumara Jivaka, the famous physician who was Buddha's contemporary, wrote the original treatise. In this case, he would have received these teaching lectures (probably in the previously mentioned form) from Buddha himself.

This form of medicine flourished during the time of King Ashoka, whose enormous realm extended from Cambodia to present-day Iran, as well as from Sri Lanka to the Himalayas. As India's Buddhist era drew to a close, these teachings reached Tibet. Here they were translated and preserved, then passed from teacher to student without interruption until this present day. These teachings were normally handed down from father to son within a family line.

However, there is also a very famous female lineage that has handed down the Tibetan medicine. This form was only changed to a certain degree with the introduction of the large medical academies. The translations were so accurate that a portion of this ancient knowledge has today been translated back into the Sanskrit (or Hindi) in order to supplement missing texts of the ancient Indian Ayurveda medicine.

Before the arrival of Buddhism in the seventh century A.D., a shamanic culture existed in Tibet—the so-called "Old Bon." This was founded approximately 500—600 B.C. by Tönpa ("teacher") Shenrab. Tönpa Shenrab came from the Zhang-Zhung area in western Tibet. He was the descendent of a rich family that was primarily occupied with ritualistic healing, herbs, astrology, and the like. The medicine of this cultural period was mainly dominated by shamanism, meaning that a healer mediated between the world of gods or demons and the sick person, attempting to balance the dissonance created by human beings. This corresponds entirely with the branch of the modern medical approach currently labeled as psychoneuroimmunology and works with the unity of body-mind-soul. However, a certain position of power for the shaman is connected with this approach (as well as for the physician in Western society), and it appears that this power was not always used for positive purposes.

This circumstance could actually be the basis of the old Tibetan custom of greeting each other with outstretched tongues. Everyone who was involved with magic and the respective magical practices, or consequently suffered (and continued to suffer) from poisoning, had a black-colored tongue! Poisoning appears to have been quite a popular method for achieving power in ancient cultures. Here is a passage from the Explanatory Tantra in the translation by Dr. Barry Clark (pg. 120): "One who has administered poison experiences a dry mouth, perspires, trembles with fear, is restless and looks in (all) directions with guilt and apprehension. Having understood the above one should henceforth refrain from giving harm to others."

The system of the Old Bon already had its own independent form of medicine. However, because there was no written language at that time, this was not recorded. Other sources claim that the Bon culture did have a written language and date the first medical treatise back to the time of Tönpa Shenrab. *The 400,000 Paths of Healing*, compiled by his son, is considered the standard work of the medical lineage of the Bon. In 1985, a copy of the block printing of the original Bon text was discovered by archeologists in eastern Tibet. In 1993, stones with an original language from Zhang-Zhung were found in the region of Ngari. These stones indicate that there had already been a written language in this area in 3000—5000 B.C. Whether or not these are fakes can probably only be clarified by the historians.

According to historical reports, there were already encounters between Indian adepts and physicians and the Tibetan culture in the second century A.D. During this time, it is said that Tibetan physicians were already trained and the first physician family line was established. Other sources date the beginning of this family line back to the fifth century.

However, the absolute turning point in the culture of Tibet took place in the seventh century A.D. under the rulership of the 32nd king of Tibet, Songtsen Gampo (617-650). He was married to a Nepalese and a Chinese princess and supported Buddhism in every imaginable form. This led to the great dissemination and acceptance of Buddhist teachings within Tibet.

Both princesses have sometimes also been considered as the emanations of the Green Tara and White Tara. Tara is viewed as the feminine representative of the mercy of all the Buddhas and is the companion of Avalokiteshvara, the Bodhisattva of compassion. He, in turn, is the "patron saint" of Tibet and manifests himself in the form of the Dalai Lama. The White Tara grants protection, peace, and a long life. The Green Tara helps in overcoming obstacles and rescues sentient beings from dangerous situations.

Under the auspices of King Songtsen Gampo, there was a lively exchange of cultures and knowledge between Tibet and India, and between Tibet and China. The scholar Thomi Sambhota was sent to India to develop a written language, and the Indian physician Damakosha, as well as the Chinese physician Hashang Mahadeva, subsequently translated medical texts into the Tibetan language. At this time, three notable physicians met at the invitation of the king: Bara Datsa (Bharad-vaja) from India, Hen Wong Hong from China, and Galeno from Persia. Together (probably in cooperation with a Tibetan physician) they wrote a summary of all their experiences under the title of *The Weapon of Invincibility*. Unfortunately, this work has been lost in the course of time.

There is some disagreement in the history books about the physician Galeno. Some think he came from Turkestan, while others point to old Persia, meaning modern-day Iran. In any case, his name permits the conclusion that he embodied the ancient Greek-Persian philosophy of medicine and that this knowledge reached Tibet through him. Incidentally, Galeno remained in Tibet as the king's personal physician and, founded a famous family dynasty under the family name of "Tsoru" in Tibet's medical history.

Physicians from the above-mentioned countries also came to Tibet under the 37th king of Tibet, Me-Ok Tsom (698-755). Hashang Mahachina (*Hashang* means physician) came from China and Biché Tsenpashila from Persia. This Persian physician also founded a medical family line, which came to be known under the name of the "Bichi line." The important Tibetan physician Chunpo Tsitsi lived during this period and the medical work *Soma Ratsa* (The Moon King) was created through the teamwork of these physicians.

Under the rulership of the 38th king of Tibet, Trison Detsen (742-796), Buddhism was proclaimed the state religion. In addition, the first medical academy was established in the year 762. Berotsana, who is probably identical with Vairocano, directed the academy. Berotsana or Vairocana was a famous translator and student of the important Indian adept Padmasambhave, who is called Guru Rinpoche (precious teacher) in Tibet. He was one of the most significant communicators of Tantric Buddhism in Tibet.

It is possible that Berotsana, in cooperation with Yuthok Yonten Goenpo the Elder (also called Yuthok Nyingma) integrated the ancient healing techniques of the Bon period into the medical works at this time. It is generally assumed that the *Gyushi*—the four fundamental medical tantras—were created during this era. Another version reports that the Indian adept Chandrananda, together with Vairocana, translated the basic texts from Sanskrit and disseminated them.

This text was concealed in a pillar of the Samye Monastery as a so-called "Treasure Text " (Tib. *terma*) so that it could be rediscovered at the appropriate time by the people suited for this purpose and thereby remain preserved for humanity.

The first medical academy, which was created on the border to Kham, had 300 students when it opened. After these students had completed the ten-year(!) period of studies, the second cycle began. The academy already had 1000 students, making it possible to do extensive research and studies thereafter. Thanks to the king's love of horses, veterinary medicine was also introduced. Through the teamwork of the Indian physician Dharmaraja, the Chinese physician Mahachina, and the Persian physician, the medical work *The Jewel Vase* (Tib. *Rinchen Bumpa*) was produced. Unfortunately, only a small portion of this medical treatise is available today.

This golden epoch for Tibet's culture was followed by a very dark period of war and repression under the ruler Langdarma (born in 842). This era continued until the year 1052. Only after this time did peace return to the Roof of the World.

The Tibetan translator Rinchen Zangpo (958-1055) lived in India for a longer period of time and brought the medical work *The Essences of the Eight Branches* (Tib. *Yenla Jaypa*) to Tibet in the later years of his life. In its content, this work corresponds very closely to Ayurvedic medicine. Yuthok Sarma (also called Yuthok Yonten Goenpo the Younger), who is considered to be one of the most outstanding physicians of all time, was also alive during this period. He came from the same family as Yuthok the Elder—but 13 generations later. On the basis of the works by Yuthok Nyingma and Berotsana (and probably also consulting the *Essences of the Eight Branches*), he compiled the fundamental medical work known to this day as the *Gyushi: the "Secret Oral Tradition of the Eight Branches of the Science of Healing,"* which is divided into four treatises.

One more important stage within Tibetan medicine is the introduction of detoxified mercury by Mahasiddha Urgyenpa (1230-1310), who traveled extensively through Pakistan, Kashmir, and the neighboring countries. The detoxified mercury constitutes a basic component of all "jewel pills," a much-praised Tibetan medicinal specialty. A very detailed collection of texts on all medical substances (materia medica)—the *Ocean of Medical Substances* (Tib. *Men Ming Gyamtso*)—also originated during this period.

Desi Sangye Gyatso (1653-1705)), the regent of the 5th Dalai Lama, founded the medical university on the iron mountain near Lhasa, Chagpori. In addition, he wrote the much-praised commentary *Blue Beryl* about the *Gyushi*. In 1627, a very extensive materia medica, *The Crystal Mirror* (Tib. *Shel Gong*, also translated as "Crystal Orb") was created by Demar Geshe. In this pharmacopoeia, a great variety of medical substances is described in very detailed form, totaling 2294 entries. His commentary on his own work, *The Crystal Rosary* (Tib. *Shel Treng*), is considered to be outstanding.

In the year 1754, his student, the 8th Situ Choeji Jungmé (1700-1774) established the Palpung Academy near his Palpung Monastery. The five branches of knowledge—defined as astrology, medicine, mathematics, poetry, and linguistics—were taught here. Along with several other monastery universities, Palpung became one of the leading academies of Tibet.

In the year 1916, the 13th Dalai Lama founded a further medical academy in the capital city of Lhasa, the Mentsee-Khang. This school was newly rebuilt as the Tibetan Institute for Medicine and Astrology in Dharamsala/northern India by the 14th Dalai Lama, Tenzin Gyatso, after his forced flight because of the Chinese occupation of Tibet. Today, the institute is once again training physicians of Tibetan medicine, runs a small affiliated hospital, and also produces most of the generally prescribed medicinal mixtures.

The venerable Chagpori Institute has also been newly founded in Darjeeling (northern India) under the direction of the outstanding Tibetan lama and physician Dr. Trogawa Rinpoche. Today it once again trains Tibetan physicians.

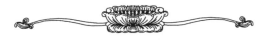

Section I

The Healthy Body

Fundamental Information
on the Three Bodily Energies

When we study Tibetan medicine, it is absolutely necessary to take a closer look at the underlying causes of reincarnation of the body-mind continuum in one form or the other.

The basic impulses of reincarnation are formed by the mental impulses that accompany each sentient being from one incarnation to the next, at least as a potential. The basic impulse is the false assumption that an independent and autonomous "self" exists. This fundamentally false perspective of reality, which can also be called basic ignorance, consequently creates the three mental poisons. These ultimately produce a total of 84,000 so-called affective emotions (causing suffering).

With the exception of completely pure beings, such as Buddhas and Bodhisattvas, who reincarnate as a voluntary decision solely based on compassion for all other beings, basic ignorance—as well as the three resulting mental poisons of desire (wishes, passions, attachments), anger (irritation, rage, hatred), and a limited perspective of reality (stupidity, closed-mindedness, apathy)—are the basis for all other beings for their respective reincarnation, as well as their associated physical, emotional, and mental abilities and/or difficulties.

This is why the three mental poisons are considered to be distant causes for illness. As previously mentioned, the absolute primary basic cause is seen to be in the false view of reality. The specified impulses encounter the so-called "Bardo body" (a type of dream body during the transition from one form of incarnation to the next) in a very extreme manner and guide it into a phenomenal world. This world corresponds with the more or less positive or negative illusions that the "Bardo body" has created from within itself.

The (mistaken) perception of this phenomenal world as the only possible "reality" intensifies insistence upon the acceptance of an independently existing "self" that is separate from everything else and exists from within itself. In the Buddhist perspective, an infinite number of "realities" exist and everything is dependent upon and resonates with all other things in this universe.

In Buddhism, the attainment of a human body is not considered to be a self-evident truth. Instead, it is seen as something of distinct value. The human incarnation offers an outstanding opportunity for perceiving the fundamental reality within one life span and thereby liberating oneself from the wheel of reincarnation and the suffering that accompanies it.

As described above, the three mental poisons form the basis for the corresponding principles of *Lung* (wind), *Tripa* (bile), and *Péken* (phlegm). These poisons exist on the material, the emotional, as well as the mental level. The Tibetan word for them is also called *nyepa*, which literally means "error."

In a Western oriented cosmology, this corresponds most closely to the idea of a basic "Males," a fundamental disposition that already exists latently, which is now awaiting its respective activation. The possibilities of this activation are explained in greater detail in the next chapter.

In the Indian system of Ayurveda, this fundamental division into three is called *tridosha*, which is composed of the energetic principles of *vata*, *pitta*, and *kapha*.

The Spagyric-alchemical view of how all things are divided into three (sal, sulphur, and mercury) can also be mentioned here as the classical-Western heritage, which is still in use today.

The anthroposophic philosophy is also based on these three principles and calls them thinking, feeling, and desiring, as well as other names. The fundamental perspective, as well as the medicinal mixtures of anthroposophic medicine, show some common elements with Eastern systems of philosophy and medicine.

The Western teaching about the development of the three germ layers (endoderm, mesoderm, and ectoderm) can also be cited as an example of this fundamental classification; and a fundamental division into three in all dynamic systems is also recognized in modern chaos research. It is assumed here that three different forces effect each other in a reciprocal action in the interference rhythm. All forms are built from these three different forces. By means of an additional feedback system, a self-controlling, dynamic self-regulating cycle is created.

But the normal situation is that one or the other of them dominates or even two or all three energies predominate at the same time. The result of this is that the corresponding errors dominate in terms of diet and behavior.

This concurs with the following analogy: The prevailing bodily energy forms a magnetic target. Now the errors, as well as the positive influences, that have the respective resonance will generally hit the target quite automatically. This results in the fact that every human being is personally responsible for recognizing that he or she is such an individually characterized "magnetic target" with the corresponding levels of resonance. Consequently, we must discover an optimal adjustment of our dietary habits and behavior, as well as our way of thinking and our attitudes. This will lead to a higher degree of "positive resonance" that hits the target, which ultimately also contributes to quicker spiritual development and liberation.

Basic Classification of Types

"Which Bodily Energy Type
Best Describes You?"

The following brief overview of the various constitutional types on the basis of their prevailing bodily energy provides a practically oriented summary of the last chapter. In addition, there is a two-part test on page 236f. with which you can determine your basic type and also discover where there may be an imbalance in your bodily energies.

You can determine which bodily energy type best describes you on the following pages.

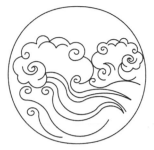

Bodily Energy Type *LUNG* (Wind)

- ○ Tall and slender
- ○ Fine body structure
- ○ Tends toward thin and dry skin
- ○ Mental alertness, quickness of mind
- ○ Tends toward sleeplessness
- ○ Tends to be worried and afraid
- ○ Likes to dance and laugh
- ○ Artistic inclinations
- ○ Loves beautiful conversations in pleasant surroundings
- ○ Tends to have complaints in lower back area
- ○ Tends to eat irregularly
- ○ Quick reactions
- ○ Tends to have a high and fine voice
- ○ Strong powers of imagination
- ○ Tends to be unconventional
- ○ Inclined to emphasize the immaterial realm
- ○ Tends toward weak nerves, twitching, unrest, etc.
- ○ Light and carefree manner
- ○ Quick ease
- ○ Strong intuition with high degree of sensitivity

- ○ Confirmation of *Lung* (wind) type

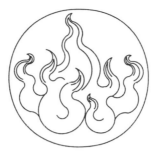

Bodily Energy Type *TRIPA* (Bile)

O Athletic, muscular build
O Medium body height
O Tends toward hot and dry skin with pigment spots
O Has no problems sleeping anywhere
O Tends toward impatience and irritation
O Loves competition
O Very motivated and goal-oriented
O High level of energy with strong dynamics
O Very direct and energetic
O Tends toward loss of self-control and sensitivity
O Is frequently "under pressure"
O Loves a cool and shady environment
O Rarely has digestive problems; can practically eat at any time and eat everything
O Tends toward complaints in upper part of body (for example, shooting headaches)
O Tends toward dominance
O Quick and vehement reactions
O Clear and strong voice
O Intense belief in self
O "Fiery" will with strong powers of assertion

O Confirmation of *Tripa* (bile) type

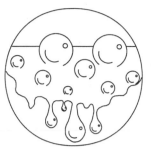

Bodily Energy Type *PÉKEN* (Phlegm)

- Tends to be short in height
- Powerful and possibly stocky build
- Tends toward large-pored and moist skin
- Very patient
- Likes to sleep and get plenty of it
- Tends to be inattentive
- Very reliable and persevering, but also slow
- Tends to be conventional
- Inclined to emphasize the material world
- Prefers reading, as well as quiet activities and hobbies
- Loves drawn-out meals
- Tends toward digestive complaints
- Loves a warm and calm environment
- Tends to be ponderous
- "Content" character
- Deep, resounding voice
- Practically oriented with inclination toward narrow perspective
- Slow reactions
- Practically oriented mental structure

- Confirmation of *Péken* (phlegm) type

The Tibetan Medicine Tree

To make it easier to understand, the Tibetan Medicine is traditionally illustrated in the form of a tree. This tree of medicine has three roots, from which nine trunks grow. Each of these continues to divide into branches and leaves, as well as blossoms and fruits on the first trunk—the results of a conscious and balanced life.

The first root
treats the object of the examination, meaning the body in its healthy and in its diseased form.

The second root
treats the diagnostic possibilities.

The third root
treats the therapeutic possibilities.

The system in this portrayal corresponds with a table of contents, from which we can get a clear and quick overview of the entire arrangement of the Medicine Tantras.

"Root of the Structure
of the Healthy and the Diseased Body"

Two trunks come from this root, from which a total of twelve branches extend. In turn, there are 88 leaves, as well as two blossoms and three fruits, on these trunks.

The 1st trunk ("the trunk of the healthy body) has 3 branches with a total of 25 leaves, as well as two blossoms and three fruits:
- Branch with bodily fluids (15 leaves)
- Branch with bodily components (7 leaves)
- Branch of the bodily excretions (3 leaves)
Two blossoms: Health and long life
Three fruits: Prosperity, happiness, and spiritual evolution

The 2nd trunk ("the trunk of the diseased body") has 9 branches with a total of 63 leaves:
- Branch of the (primary) causes (3 leaves)
- Branch of the immediate causes (4 leaves)
- Branch of the entrances of illness (6 leaves)
- Branch of location (3 leaves)
- Branch of the passageways (circulatory paths) (15 leaves)
- Branch of the times of origin (9 leaves)
- Branch of the deadly results (9 leaves)
- Branch of the side effects (12 leaves)
- Branch of the categories (hot and cold) (2 leaves)

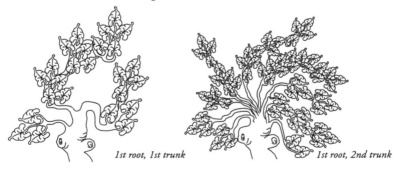

1st root, 1st trunk   1st root, 2nd trunk

"Root of the Diagnostic Techniques"

Three trunks come from this root, from which a total of eight branches extend. In turn, there are 38 leaves on these branches.

The 1st trunk ("trunk of visual examination") has 2 branches with a total of 6 leaves:
- Branch of visual examination of the tongue (3 leaves)
- Branch of visual examination of the urine (3 leaves)

The 2nd trunk ("trunk of palpation") has 3 branches with a total of 3 leaves:
- Branch of pulse examination for *Lung*/wind (1 leaf)
- Branch of pulse examination for *Tripa*/bile (1 leaf)
- Branch of pulse examination for *Péken*/phlegm (1 leaf)

The 3rd trunk ("trunk of questioning") has 3 branches with a total of 29 leaves:
- Branch of activating causes (3 leaves)
- Branch of symptoms (23 leaves)
- Branch of living habits and eating habits (3 leaves)

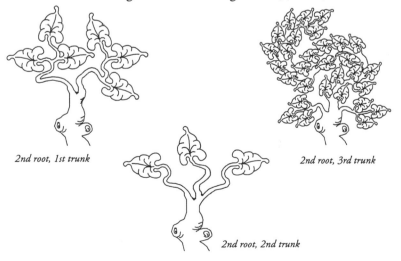

2nd root, 1st trunk

2nd root, 3rd trunk

2nd root, 2nd trunk

"Root of Therapeutic Process"

Four trunks come from this root, upon which a total of 27 branches shoot off. In turn, there are 98 leaves on these branches.

The 1st trunk (trunk of nutrition) has 6 branches with a total of 35 leaves.
- Branch of foods for *Lung* diseases (10 leaves)
- Branch of beverages for *Lung* diseases (4 leaves)
- Branch of foods for *Tripa* diseases (7 leaves)
- Branch of beverages for *Tripa* diseases (5 leaves)
- Branch of foods for *Péken* diseases (6 leaves)
- Branch of beverages for *Péken* diseases (3 leaves)

The 2nd trunk (trunk of living habits) has a total of 3 branches with 6 leaves.
- Branch of living habits *for Lung* diseases (2 leaves)
- Branch of living habits for *Tripa* diseases (2 leaves)
- Branch of living habits for *Péken* diseases (2 leaves)

The 3rd trunk (trunk of remedies) has a total of 15 branches with 50 leaves.
- Branch of the taste of *Lung* remedies (3 leaves)
- Branch of the taste of *Tripa* remedies (3 leaves)
- Branch of the taste of *Péken* remedies (3 leaves)

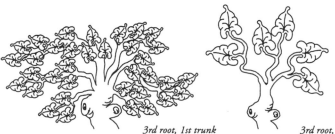

3rd root, 1st trunk   *3rd root, 2nd trunk*

- Branch of powers of medicines for *Lung* remedies (3 leaves)
- Branch of powers of medicines for *Tripa* remedies (3 leaves)
- Branch of powers of medicines for *Péken* remedies (3 leaves)
- Branch of pacification through soups for *Lung* (3 leaves)
- Branch of pacification through medicinal oils/medicinal butter for *Lung* (3 leaves)
- Branch of pacification through decoctions for *Tripa* (4 leaves)
- Branch of pacification through powders for *Tripa* (4 leaves)
- Branch of pacification through pills for *Péken* (2 leaves)
- Branch of pacification through calcinated powders for *Péken* (5 leaves)
- Branch of cleansing evacuation through suppositories for *Lung* (3 leaves)
- Branch of cleansing evacuation through purgation for *Tripa* (3 leaves)
- Branch of cleansing evacuation through emesis for *Péken* (3 leaves)

The 4th trunk (trunk of accessory therapies) has 3 branches with a total of 7 leaves.
- Branch of accessory therapies for *Lung* (2 leaves = oil massage; moxa/cauterization)
- Branch of accessory therapies for *Tripa* (3 leaves = sudorifics; venesection and cold fomentation)
- Branch of accessory therapies for *Péken* (2 leaves = hot fomentation; moxa)

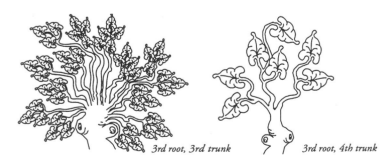

3rd root, 3rd trunk   *3rd root, 4th trunk*

The Elements and Their Classifications

According to the Tibetan standpoint, our universe is made of the five elements of *space, air, fire, water,* and *earth*. Tibetan cosmology gives a detailed description of how each of these elements comes from the previous one in this series. As a result, the formation of all "things" is begun. However, there is no valuation related to this since all of the elements are equally required for the formation of the universe. Since all things—including human beings—in this universe are formed from the same five elements, it is possible to make an analysis through the respective composition of these elements. By means of intellectual perception, intuition, and Tibetan medicine's centuries of experience, deviations in a human being's energy balance can be recognized. The respective appropriate form of treatment can then be selected on this basis. Consequently, healing in Tibetan medicine occurs through the balancing of the elements in a person's state of individual harmony. This is not intended to be seen in a purely chemical-material sense. For a more comprehensive understanding of this concept, it is necessary to look at the nature of the elements themselves.

An "element" is—as the name already implies—part of a whole. This means that there are no pure elements that exist on their own: The corresponding exceptions confirm the rule. All things contain each of the elements in various combined proportions or energy balances, which also determines the respective form of manifestation. So we must differentiate between the manner of manifestation or the dynamic processes of an element that take place at this moment and its fundamental nature. This inquiry occurs through an intuitive, as well as through an analytical approach. The facts of the analytical approach can be found in this chapter or in more detailed form in a book on chemistry or physics.

By approaching this in an intuitive manner, it is possible to encounter the nature of the respective element in a "heartfelt" manner. We can listen to the murmuring of a stream or look into an evening fire. How does a piece of earth, a tree, or a stone feel in your hands? What effect does the wind have on a lake? What type of ripples occur during which season? What happens to the fire when the wind blows? All human beings are familiar with these kinds of experiences. So it is possible for every individual to take the elements to heart by simply letting this happen, without any exertion—because we are all made of these elements ourselves!

When we have comprehended both the analytical as well as the sensory form of examination, all the possible combinations of the process dynamics in their respective expressions and forms of manifestation will then result quite automatically. The game of life is a dance of the elements—one of the fundamental keys to understanding Tibetan medicine lies in the holistic comprehension of these dynamic interdependencies.

As already stated, each human being is composed of the same elements as the universe itself—only in differing proportions. The basic laws can then be recognized in both the microscopic (or microcosmic) framework and the macroscopic (or macrocosmic) framework. One Branch of Tibetan physician's training consists of learning astrology. The reason for this is that without the fundamental cosmic state of resonance, the smaller depiction of the cosmos—the human being—cannot be understood (for more about biorhythmic-planetary influences, also see *Non-Visible Forces*, page 79f.)

In order to clearly recognize the composition of the elements in the microcosmic framework of medicinal plants, minerals, etc., the Tibetan system of medicine has developed the perception and differentiation of tastes as the basic parameter in an extraordinarily detailed manner. This will be described in a later chapter (see page 106f.)

Should the reader already be familiar with the Chinese theory of elements, here is how it differs from the Tibetan:

TIBETAN/CHINESE THEORY OF ELEMENTS

Tibetan		Chinese
Wind (Air)	corresponds to	Wood
Fire	corresponds to	Fire
Earth	corresponds to	Earth + Iron (Metal)
Water	corresponds to	Water
Space	no correlation	

THE ELEMENTS HAVE THE FOLLOWING
FUNDAMENTAL ASSOCIATIONS:

Wind . . . corresponds to . . . Movement, growth, inspiration, creativity

Fire . . . . corresponds to . . . Energy, heat, passion

Earth . . . corresponds to . . . Solid matter, stability, sense of reality

Water . . . corresponds to . . . Cohesion (adhesive power; attraction within matter), passivity, cold, receptivity, calm

Space . . . . Permeates all the elements and gives them room to develop

Moving inspiration in the form of air permeates the fundamental living space. Fire allows this thought to mature and grow through warmth. Water holds it together and the earth gives it stability in a formative manner.

Among other things, you can find further associations and qualities in the following chapter on bodily energies and their corresponding subcategories.

THE CLASSIFICATION OF THE THREE BODILY
PRINCIPLES WITH THE ELEMENTS:

Lung (Wind) . . . . corresponds to . . . . Air + Space

Tripa (Bile) . . . . corresponds to . . . . Fire

Péken (Phlegm) . . . . corresponds to . . . . Earth + Water

The classification of the tastes and the powers of medicine can be found on page 106. You can read about the reciprocal relationship of the elements with each other in the chapter on pulse diagnosis (see page 147f.)

The Three Bodily Energies Lung (Wind), Tripa (Bile), and Péken (Phlegm), with Their Subcategories

The three fundamental bodily energies or principles of being are *Lung* (wind), *Tripa* (bile), and *Péken* (phlegm). As already stated above, their emotional or mental equivalents form the causes for reincarnation. In the following section, their fundamental analogies and qualities, as well as their physical subcategories, including the mode of action, will be portrayed. The respective chapters will discuss in detail the characteristics of the bodily energies in terms of the basic constitution, diet, etc.

རླུང།

Lung (Wind)

Lung/wind is very basically associated with the mind in the Tibetan perspective. It is therefore considered the basic cause of all diseases. Many of the illnesses classified as "psychosomatic" in the West have a strong *Lung* character. Although wind is generally cool and is therefore related to the illnesses that are classified as "cold," its flexibility is also capable of fanning the fire. As a result, it is a contributing factor to so many illnesses. In the ancient Greek humoral pathology as well, the *pneuma* (Greek for "spirit") represents the mental aspect, along with other aspects. The bodily energy *Lung* symbolizes all of the dynamic processes in the body and represents the element of air. Although the bodily energies are always present in the entire body, the main location of *Lung* is described as being in the heart, as well as in the lower portion of the body (below the navel). *Lung* effects the structuring of the body, as well as inhalation and exhalation. It moves the blood in the blood vessels and serves to sustain the body through these activities. *Lung* is generally responsible for the clarity of the sensory organs.

Lung (wind) has these basic characteristics:

- ■ flexible/mobile
- ■ coarse
- ■ cool (to cold)

- ■ subtle (fine)
- ■ light
- ■ hard (firm)

The characteristic "subtle" refers to the possibility that *Lung* (wind) has of permeating everything. The characteristic "hard" refers to an opposing force. Going against the wind could be used as an example of this: It is "hard" to make progress against the strength of the wind.

The Bodily Energy *Lung* (Wind) Is Divided into Five Subcategories:

1. The Life-Sustaining Wind

Its seat is on the crown of the head. This wind circulates from its seat to the middle of the chest area. It is responsible for the swallowing of solid and fluid foods, for inhalation and exhalation, for spitting, for crying, for sneezing and nose blowing, as well as for repeating and burping. In addition, it provides clear senses, lucid mental functioning, and powers of concentration. It offers the physical basis for the mental continuum and is therefore the "interface" of the body and mind, which it holds together. Since it also advances the ingested food through the esophagus to the stomach, the following saying applies to this type of wind: eating and drinking holds the body and soul together.

2. The Ascending Wind

Its seat is found in the chest at the level of the breastbone. It primarily moves in the areas of the nose and the tongue, as well as in the throat. In the latter area, it acts in interrelation with the life-sustaining wind. It is responsible for speaking, promotes a clear memory and alertness, provides bodily strength, supports initiative, and furnishes strong charisma and a clear skin color.

3. The Pervading Wind

Its seat is found in the heart, especially in the so-called "life channel." However, it passes through and permeates the entire body. It is responsible for physical motion, for the stretching and bending of the limbs, and for the opening and closing of the body openings (such as the mouth and eyes). Almost all movements of the body are based on it.

4. The Fire-Accompanying Wind

Another name for this wind is: "the fire-like equalizing wind." Its seat is found in the lower portion of the stomach. It wanders through all of the hollow organs (stomach, small intestine, large intestine, gallbladder, urinary bladder, and life vessel). It is responsible for digestion to the extent that it separates what has been ingested into nutriments and eliminatory substances. Furthermore, it is partially responsible for the maturation of the bodily components.

5. The Downward Voiding Wind

This wind is also called "the downwards driving wind" or "the downward clearing wind." Its seat is in the genital area, as well as in the area of the anus—both are so-called "secret areas." It circulates in the large intestine, in the urinary bladder, the genitals, and the thighs. It controls the retention or the ejaculation of the semen, the menstrual blood, the stool, and the urine, as well as the fetus during birth.

Tripa (Bile)

The bodily energy *Tripa* is—as can easily be seen in the characteristics of anger and rage that effect it—responsible for the heat principle in the body. All fire aspects, meaning the fundamental thermodynamics, as well as the body's nutrition and digestion, form its main area of activity; *Tripa*/bile makes sure that we feel hunger and thirst. The associated element is fire. *Tripa* is also responsible for body heat, gives us courage, and provides clear skin and positive charisma. The intellect is also dependent upon it. The main location of this bodily energy is said to be "between the navel and the heart." In the Galenic humor pathology, the bile is subdivided twice. In Tibetan medicine, the principles of "bile and blood" are differentiated. All of the diseases that are classified as "hot" are related to an imbalance of *Tripa*/bile.

The fundamental characteristics of the bodily energy Tripa (bile) are:

- hot
- biting-spicy
- light
- oily

- quickly acting
- (slightly) purgative
- malodorous
- liquid

The Bodily Energy *Tripa* (bile) Is Divided into Five Subcategories:

1. The Digestive Bile

Its seat is found in the center of the digestive tract between the food that has not yet been digested and what has already been digested. It can be equated with the "digestive heat" and therefore is extremely important for maintaining a healthy body. Its task is to digest the ingested food, as well as separating the nourishing substances from the excess, which means the cleansed from the non-cleansed material. It provides the body heat and supports all of the other four types of *Tripa*/bile. The digestive bile generally increases physical strength.

2. The Coloring Bile

Other terms in use for this are "the color-transforming bile" or "the color-regulating bile." Its seat is in the liver. The coloring bile is responsible for the transformation of the colors in the nutriment, as well as the other bodily constituents. Through it, the blood becomes red, the bile flow becomes yellow, etc. The color of the skin also depends upon this type of *Tripa*/bile.

3. The Accomplishing Bile

This type of bile can also be called the "realizing," "stimulating," or "determining bile." Its seat is found in the heart. It furnishes people with courage, intelligence, and willpower, therefore providing the necessary powers of assertion and self-confidence in achieving the corresponding wishes and goals. In the negative sense, however, this can develop into an overestimation of one's own abilities and pride.

4. The Visual Bile

This bile has its seat in the eyes and makes it possible for people to see external objects.

5. The Skin-and-Complexion Clearing Bile

The seat of this type of bile is in the skin. It provides the color and complexion of the skin and its elasticity, as well as an individual's clear charisma—which is the result of this.

བད་ཀན།

Péken (Phlegm)

The bodily energy *Péken* (phlegm) corresponds with the fluid aspect of the body and therefore represents the water element. All bodily fluids are dependent upon phlegm, which is responsible for the lubrication of the entire body (including the joints). As a result, it furnishes the connections within the body, as well as its softness and elasticity. It is responsible for all of the moist and wet factors of the body. *Péken* (phlegm) also provides for the firmness of the body and the mind (in the form of patience). In this manner, it creates a stable foundation and corresponds in this aspect to the earth element. Within humoral pathology, its classification would be *phlegma*. The desire to sleep also results from this bodily energy. On the basis of the stated characteristics, it becomes clear why it is also related to hazy, foggy, and dull senses. It then has a heavy and static character. The level "above the heart" is considered the main location of this bodily energy.

The bodily energy Péken (phlegm) has the following basic characteristics:

- cool
- heavy
- blunt
- oily
- gentle

- smooth
- static
- adhesive (sticky)
- solid (stable)
- slowly acting

The Bodily Energy *Péken* (Phlegm) Is Also Divided into Five Subcategories

1. The Supporting Phlegm

Its seat is in the chest, primarily along the breastbone. It supports all the other four types of phlegm and is responsible for the water equilibrium, meaning the general level of moisture in the body.

2. The Decomposing Phlegm

This type of phlegm is also called "mixing phlegm" or "kneading phlegm." Its location is in the upper portion of the digestive tract, exactly at the point where the undigested food collects—primarily in the upper section of the stomach. For the food to slowly move into the stomach, with the help of the "supporting phlegm," it is "held" at the junction between the esophagus and the entrance to the stomach, down to the first section of the stomach. The "decomposing phlegm" then causes the mixing of solid and liquid foods. Then it decomposes them, which should be seen as an important stage in the separation of food within the digestive tract.

3. The Experiencing Phlegm

This is also called "the phlegm that makes the experience of tasting." Its seat is in the tongue and cavity of the mouth. It provides for the perception of the six different tastes: sweet, sour, salty, bitter, hot, and astringent. (For more on this topic, see *The Taste Type*, on page 106 f.).

4. The Satisfying Phlegm

This has its seat in the head area and satisfies the senses. As a result, we consider tones as pleasant sounds, smells as good smells, tastes as good tastes, and see beauty in the objects that we perceive to be beautiful, etc.

5. The Connecting Phlegm

Its location is found in the joints, where it creates the connection within the joints so that they can be bent and stretched.

Summary: The three basic energies can be understood as the physiological and biochemical processes in the bodily area. *Lung* (wind) is classified with the activities of the nervous system, as well as the metabolism in general. *Tripa* (bile) is associated more with the catabolic (= decomposing) metabolic processes; *Péken* (phlegm) is associated more with the anabolic (= structuring) metabolic processes.

When the three bodily energies are found in the corresponding quantity in their respective seats (location), health and balance are provided. This means that imbalances and disturbances of the bodily energies can occur through the factors of increase or decrease in the quantities, as well as through a shift in location.

The Seven Bodily Constituents

A total of seven bodily constituents form the body, thereby sustaining it. Each of these bodily constituents exists in a precisely defined amount. Disturbances and imbalances can therefore result from an increase or decrease of these basic substances.

According to the perspective of Tibetan medicine, these basic substances of the body are formed through the metabolic processes triggered by the ingested food. In this process, one *nourishing essence*

49

and one *waste product* is produced respectively. This means that one cleansed and one non-cleansed portion is created. With the exception of the waste products produced at the very beginning of this metabolic process (feces and urine), both portions are always fundamentally important for sustaining the body.

When there is a decrease in the quality of the respective essences, disturbances can also occur in the form of illnesses. The successive metabolic chains of the cleansed essences, as well as the waste products, will be described later in this chapter. The principle of digestive heat, together with the digestive process, will be illuminated first.

The Digestive Heat

In the texts of Tibetan medicine, four or seven subcategories of digestive heat are described. However, the digestive heat can be virtually equated with "digestive bile" for our purposes. This metabolic heat forms the basis for the entire thermic regulation of the body, as well as the actual digestive process. If the digestive heat is too weak, a large portion of the ingested food will be eliminated in an undigested form. The result is that part of the food will be wasted through poor separation and utilization, which additionally burdens the body. This may be expressed in the form of flatulence, etc. Furthermore, certain symptoms of deficiency will develop in the course of time because of lacking nutrients when the digestive heat is weak. Consequently, just taking additional nutritional supplements, vitamins, etc., without simultaneously supporting the digestive heat is rather pointless in the long run.

Through the warm and light foods described in *Dietary Habits*, on page 98ff., the digestive heat can be protected and supported. According to the Tibetan perspective, this is the precondition for a healthy and long life. However, the digestive heat can also become too active. Then it attacks the bodily constituents and practically "burns" them, which can also lead to symptoms of deficiency and a general emaciation of the body in the long run.

The digestive heat fulfills the following factors:

- Provides heat (general thermic regulation of the body)
- Separates nutriments (the essence) from excess matter (waste substances).
- Drives excess matter out of the digestive area after digestion has occurred.
- Prevents undigested substances from reaching the passageways of digested food.
- Increases bodily constituents
- Responsible for a good skin color, as well as clear and strong charisma
- Provides physical strength.

The effects of a dominance of one bodily energy on the digestive heat

When there is an excess of *Lung* (wind), the digestive heat will be unstable.

When there is an excess of *Tripa* (bile), the digestive heat will be accelerated and overactive.

When there is an excess of *Péken* (phlegm), the digestive heat will be slowed down.

When there is an excess of a combination of *Lung/Tripa* (wind/bile), the digestive heat will be very vehement and very active.

When there is an excess of a combination of *Tripa/Péken* (bile/phlegm), the digestive heat will be in an average state.

When there is an excess of a combination of *Lung/Péken* (wind/phlegm), the digestive heat will be weak.

DOMINANCE OF BODILY ENERGY AND DIGESTIVE HEAT

Excess of	Effect on Digestive Heat
Lung	Unstable, irregular
Tripa	Accelerated, overactive
Péken	Slowed down
Lung/Tripa	Very active and vehement
Tripa/Péken	Average
Lung/Péken	Weak

If all three bodily energies are in a balanced state of flow, the digestive heat will also be in an optimal condition.

The Digestive Process

In the Tibetan texts, the entire digestive process takes place in the stomach. However, we can assume that this is the general term for the entire gastrointestinal tract—meaning the stomach, duodenum, small intestine, and a portion of the large intestine. Moreover, the location of a certain bodily energy does not mean fixation but rather a dominance in this special area of the body. The Tibetan word for "digesting" means "melting." During the digestive process, the character of the chyme (mass of partly digested food) changes—and therefore also the proportion of the elements. According to the Tibetan approach, we could say that "the taste changes" (see *The Types of Tastes,* page 106f.) As depicted in detail further below, the entire digestive system activates and intensifies itself as soon as it is set into motion. This means that:

1. Phlegm produces more phlegm
2. Bile produces more bile
3. Wind produces more wind

We can compare this process in part with the Western system of tissue hormones.

1. The absorbed food and drink is moved from the esophagus down into the stomach by the life-sustaining wind. The mixing phlegm is located in the upper section of the stomach. It is responsible for mixing the solid and liquid portions of the ingested foods. The fluid portions contribute to the decomposition of the food, and the oily portions of the solid food provide the corresponding softness or softening of the chyme. During this phase, the elements of earth and water increase, which means that the bodily energy of *Péken* (phlegm) increases within the entire body. This also applies to the mixing phlegm, which means that the digestive process sus-

tains and accelerates itself. The chyme becomes sweet and foamy as a result. This process last about one-half hour, but it may take up to two hours.

2. Now the digestive bile is stirred up by the fire-accompanying wind, which leads to the "boiling" and the first division of the chyme within the stomach. This is described as the "fire under a pot with medicine" in Tibetan medicine. During this phase, the elements of fire and earth increase, which leads to an intensification of the *Tripa* (bile) bodily energy within the entire body. The chyme becomes hot and sour as a result. This process lasts between one-half and one-and-a-half hours after food intake, but may possibly take up to four hours.

3. In the concluding phase, the nutritious essence is separated from the excess matter. This occurs through the fire-accompanying wind. The chyme becomes bitter as a result and the bodily energy of *Lung* (wind) increases throughout the entire body—as well as the fire-accompanying wind—on the basis of its own activity. This process usually lasts somewhere between one-and-a-half and four hours after food intake, but can also take up to six hours.

Since the body consists of the five elements and these five elements are also contained in the ingested food, they can be supplied to the body through the digestive process. This leads to sustaining the bodily functions. This process must also be understood in the qualitative sense: Denatured food cannot supply the body with a highly effective quality of elements. They only strain the digestive heat in a needless manner and burden the digestive tract unnecessarily. The 100% absorption of the digested food, or the nutriment essence that has developed from it, forms the basis for sustaining good health.

PROCESS OF THE DIGESTIVE PHASES

| Food/ Drink | → | are conveyed to the stomach by the "life-sustaining wind" |

Up to approx. ¹/2 hour after food intake
it is mixed by the "mixing phlegm";
the chyme becomes sweet and foamy,
the *Péken* in the entire body is increased.

Approx. ¹/2 to 1¹/2 hours after food intake
the "digesting bile" is stirred up by the
"fire-accompanying wind";
the chyme becomes hot and sour;
the *Tripa* in the entire body is increased.

Approx. 1¹/2 hours after food intake
the nutriment essence is separated from the excess matter
by the "fire-accompanying wind";
the chyme becomes bitter;
the *Lung* in the entire body is increased.

The Creation of the Bodily Components

After the chyme has been digested in the manner described above, it is separated in the small intestine into the cleansed nutriment essence and an uncleansed portion. This occurs in the same way as in the above-described digestive process—through mixing, digesting, and separating. This procedure is basically emulated in all of the further processes that create the bodily constituents. The uncleansed portion is divided into fluid and solid matter. The fluid portions are excreted as urine and the solid portions as feces. The cleansed nourishing essence travels to the liver through the nine essence-transporting channels.

Mainly through heat and the above-mentioned processes, this nutriment essence is additionally developed and "ripened" in the *liver;* the cleansed portion is transformed into blood. Blood is an essential component of all bodily processes and serves as communication within the body, among other things. The resulting uncleansed portion supports the decomposing phlegm during the first phase of digestion.

In the *blood,* the essences are ripened and the cleansed portion is turned into musculature. The uncleansed portion is transported to the gallbladder as bile. In the diagnosis, this substance can later be partially used in the form of "albumen" in the urine.

The essence is ripened in the *musculature* and the cleansed portion is transformed into fatty tissue and cartilage. The uncleansed portion is excreted through the nine orifices of the body. This occurs, for example, in the form of secretion at the edges of the eyes in the morning or the earwax, and so forth

In the *fatty tissue,* the essence is developed to maturation and the cleansed portion is transformed into bone. The uncleansed portion becomes perspiration and sebum or an oily component of the body that can be wiped off.

In the *bones,* the essence is ripened and the cleansed portion is transformed into bone marrow. The uncleansed portion becomes body hair, teeth, fingernails, and toenails.

In the *bone marrow,* the essence is developed to maturity and the cleansed portion is transformed into the regenerative fluids of *semen* or *ovum.* The uncleansed portion becomes skin and stools, as well as the basic solid oil components of the body. These solid oil components provide (among other things) an "oiliness" in the skin that is very valued in Tibetan medicine. By the conversion into or the excretion as feces this also gets influenced.

The cleansed portion of the regenerative fluids—also called the "white and the red element"—is transformed into the life fluid. The *life fluid* represents the basis and the quintessence of life, the purest of all essences. In Tantric writings, its seat is said to be in the heart (for example, in the life channel). But the life fluid's inherent strength fills the entire body and gives the body its radiant power and luminous appearance.

The uncleansed portion of the regenerative fluids are transformed into reproductive fluids, meaning the seminal fluid and the ovum, the basis of physical life. Its seat is in the ovaries or the testicles.

In the sense of an essential bodily basis for procreation, this corresponds to the "heart," meaning the center. Since there is no concept of hormones in Tibetan medicine, this would be a very interesting way of looking at the Western terms in order to classify them better.

The entire process of these assimilations takes about six to a maximum of seven days. So most foods require about a week to be transformed into vital fluid.

However, there are certain foods and remedies, such as the so-called "fertility medicine" or aphrodisiacs (see *Rejuvenation and the Process of Essence-Extraction,* on page 229f.), which pass through this process in some hours or even one hour .

Almost all other Tibetan remedies pass through this cycle within a maximum of 24 hours, whereby they develop a special effectiveness in each of the individual stages mentioned above.

On the other hand, there are also substances (for example, certain poisons) whose effects are delayed for up to one year.

CREATION OF THE BODILY CONSTITUENTS

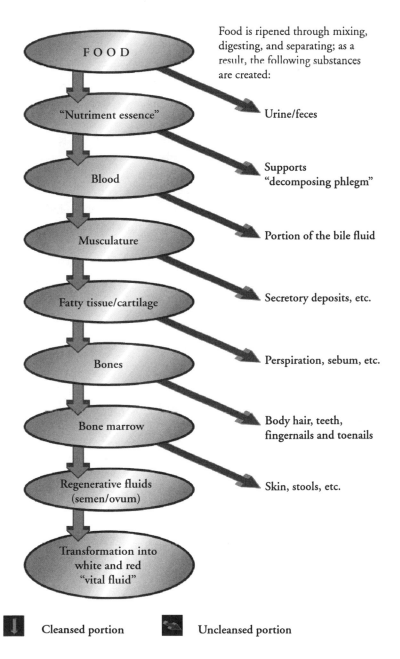

Food is ripened through mixing, digesting, and separating; as a result, the following substances are created:

FOOD

"Nutriment essence" → Urine/feces

Blood → Supports "decomposing phlegm"

Musculature → Portion of the bile fluid

Fatty tissue/cartilage → Secretory deposits, etc.

Bones → Perspiration, sebum, etc.

Bone marrow → Body hair, teeth, fingernails and toenails

Regenerative fluids (semen/ovum) → Skin, stools, etc.

Transformation into white and red "vital fluid"

Cleansed portion   Uncleansed portion

The Bodily Excretions

The branch of the bodily excretions on the main branch above the healthy body includes the factors of feces, urine, and perspiration. These are the possible ways the body can once again eliminate the non-absorbable substances in a solid or fluid form. If these excretions do not occur to an adequate degree, the body cannot free itself from the corresponding toxins. Disorders of the bodily energies will then occur.

An increase of feces can lead to constipation and a decrease can lead to diarrhea. Both of these conditions are frequently related to an imbalance of the bodily energy *Lung* (wind). Insufficient voiding of the urine can, among other things, lead to a reduction of the body coloration. Normal sweating is seen as an extremely helpful situation in Tibetan medicine since it ensures good functioning of the skin.

When an inadequate amount of sweating takes place, the skin tends to break and peel off. When there is an excess of perspiration, skin diseases may occur. Technically speaking, the body hair, as well as the toenails and fingernails, are considered to be excretory products. However, since they do not produce disorders, they are usually just seen as indicating diagnostic factors.

When the factors of the bodily excretions, the bodily constituents, as well as the bodily energies are in a balanced state of equilibrium, the result will be health and the body will blossom. If there is a disruption within the balance of these three factors, illness results.

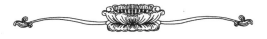

Section II

The Diseased Body

The Origin of Disease

The following analogy is made in terms of the difference or the change between the first and the second branch on the first root of the Medicine Tree: "The body in its healthy state is like water—the body in a diseased state is like ice."

This comparison is meant to show that the harmonic flow within the balance of the basic bodily substances, the bodily excretions, as well as the bodily energies, has lost its equilibrium. The comparison with ice would best apply to a cold or chronic disease, where the balance has become stagnant. For a hot or an acute disease, we could use this analogy to say that the water has turned to steam. What are the causes of this state of disharmony?

The **basic cause** of all suffering, and therefore of all diseases, is a false view of reality. This means that the body and mind become associated with a presumably independent "ego" (or "self") that exists from within itself.

We should perhaps ask where this "ego" has its actual physical seat since neither the yogis nor the neurosurgeons have ever been able to find it. And how independent is this "ego" actually? Would it possible that this "ego" can only exist in the interlinking, the synchronicity, and the resonance with all of the other "egos" or all the other elements of this universe?

To answer this (and many other) questions, Tantric science has created precisely defined instructions for experimentation within one's own body-mind continuum. With these meditation exercises, it is possible for every individual to start out on the search for answers.

In Tibetan mental training, these correlations are classically illustrated by means of a rainbow. The fundamental cause of this natural phenomenon is the sun with its rays and the triggering conditions are the raindrops. Since the raindrops fall in the direction opposite to the sun's rays, so to speak, they can be diffracted and consequently reflect the light in a certain way, which leads to the formation of the rainbow. We can see that this is a fleeting manifestation as soon as the sun is covered by a cloud or the rain stops: The previously "real" appearance of the rainbow then disappears immediately. This means that the rainbow is neither independent nor does it exist on its own.

In the same way, the "ego" is also just a phenomenon that does not exist independently. Its appearance in the material world is based on causes and triggering conditions. These may be, for example, very strong feelings, deeply rooted habits, thoughts, etc. Ultimately, the nature of the "ego" is pure emptiness, whereby "emptiness" should in no way be equated with "nothingness." In Tibetan Buddhism, emptiness is equated with an infinite space without a center and without limitation. This space is also associated with a "knowing radiance". The deepest comprehension and internalization of the fact that there is a basically non-existing "ego" leads to the lighting up of this knowing luminosity—in other words: enlightenment.

Disease is also something that does not exist from within itself, nor does it exist independently. The manifestation of diseases depends upon ignorance as the basic cause. Moreover, the primary generating causes are attachment, rejection, and apathy, as well as the direct conditions of accumulation and increase through season, improper diet, and improper behavior patterns, etc.

Fundamental ignorance leads to the creation of a total of 84,000 afflictive emotions. These correspond in turn with a total of 84,000 different diseases. They can be combined into 1616 diseases, which can be concentrated to 404 diseases. This can once again be reduced to a total of 101 primary diseases on the basis of imbalances of the bodily energies.

The Tibetans are masters at the art of perfect classifications. In the classical texts, the various disorders are divided according to many different aspects. This has the advantage that an illness can be seen and understood not only in a schematic-linear one-sided way, but also from a great variety of perspectives.

The Distant Causes of Disease

Above all, the three fundamental mental poisons of attachment (greed), anger (hatred), and apathy (obliviousness) are important for our consideration.

These three mental poisons lead directly to the formation of the three corresponding bodily energies *Lung* (wind), *Tripa* (bile), and *Péken* (phlegm). This is why they are called the distant or primary generating causes for disease. For the formation of the individual constitutional type the factors of the diet and behavior of the mother during pregnancy as well as the quality of sperm and ovum are important, too.

This is not necessarily the cause for the formation of illnesses produced by karma. However, the latent basic pattern that is shared in the mind continuum leads to resonance toward the corresponding bodily energy. Consequently, this potential is developed on the physical level.

However, for this potential to ripen it usually requires additional conditions: In the physical-emotional-mental sense, it is possible to influence how intensively and at which level these latent seeds will have an effect.

In the teaching and meditation pictures of the Tibetan medicine *thangkas*, these three distant causes are illustrated by the following animals:

Lung/wind:	Red rooster
Tripa/bile:	Green snake
Péken/phlegm:	Black pig

Other portrayals use the symbolism of a couple engaged in physical love, which leads to the creation of *Lung*. The picture of two men fist-fighting is used for the generation of *Tripa* and a sleeping person is depicted to represent the bodily energy of *Péken*.

The formation of the bodily energies through the three basic mental poisons

Bodily energy	is formed by:
Lung/wind	desire, attachment
Tripa/bile	annoyance, anger, rage, hatred
Péken/phlegm	apathy, narrow-mindedness

The Immediate Causes of Disease

The following are seen as the immediate causes or additional factors for triggering disease. These factors include both the illnesses caused by karma and those acquired in this life through the disruption of the bodily energies:

- the seasonal changes
- the diet and behavior patterns, as well as
- the so-called non-visible forces.

Each of these factors can be either

- too strong
- too weak or
- unnaturally expressed

and then lead to disorders or imbalances within the bodily harmony. Examples of these behavior patterns may be too many impressions affecting the organism through excessive television-watching or an imbalance in the bodily energies because of constantly listening to loud music. In terms of the diet, an unnatural addiction to sweets or spicy foods, etc. may exist and lead to a corresponding imbalance (see *General Behavior Patterns,* page 89f., and *Dietary Habits,* page 98f.).

The **acumulation** of a bodily energy always occurs at its own respective location. This is a natural process that corresponds with the elemental nature of the prevailing energies, such as the season, in resonance with the respective body principle. Only when the associated location is completely filled with the corresponding bodily energy does this begin to overflow into the location of another bodily energy.

For this purpose, it requires additional factors such as heat or cold. At this point in time at the latest, this overflowing appears as a disorder of the *humores* or as a manifestation of an illness. When such imbalances occur, the body shows a natural tendency toward balancing dietary habits and behavior patterns. The inner wisdom of the body will then—at least until the occurrence of an illness—have the tendency of choosing the dietary habits and behavior patterns with effective qualities that oppose the disease (also see *Seasonal Changes,"* page 72f.)

However, this instinctive wisdom of the body that is inherent to all human beings in a natural way appears to be increasingly less present. The reasons for this are the prevailing degenerated dietary habits and behavior patterns (such as excessive consumption of sugar, luxury foods, and television) in Western industrial societies. Above all, children who grow up in such an unnatural environment are not even able to develop this natural behavior any more. From the standpoint of Tibetan medicine, these children are constantly exposed to an excess of certain types of tastes, sensory impressions, etc. If opposing measures are not introduced early enough, corresponding diseases will inevitably occur. Although it may very well be a natural sign of the body when it demands something sweet, whether this desire is then satisfied with a spoon of propolis, honey or the like—or with iced cupcakes—does very much make a difference in the long run!

If you would like to stay healthy, during the corresponding times be sure to not support the qualities of this phase of acumulation. Instead, provide the appropriate balance through the opposite dietary habits and behavior patterns. If an excessive acumulation has already occurred, the manifestations of an illness can possibly be pacified through the opposite factors.

Fundamental Factors for Development and Pacification of Disease

Each of the three bodily energies is classified with a specific body area as the main location. *Lung*/wind is primarily found in the area below the navel, *Tripa*/bile is primarily found between the navel and the diaphragm, and *Péken*/phlegm is primarily found above the diaphragm.

THE SEAT OF LUNG, TRIPA, AND PÉKEN

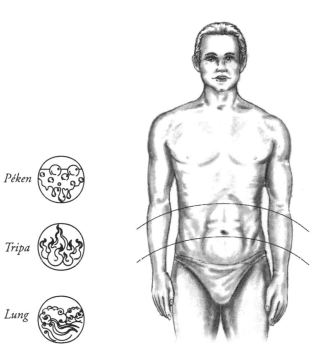

Péken

Tripa

Lung

There are fundamental factors for the increase of each of these three bodily energies, for the manifestation of the corresponding imbalance, as well as the respective disease and its pacification. All of the effective qualities mentioned can be related to the behavior patterns and the dietary habits, as well as the inner and outer treatment possibilities.

Causes of increase:
- *Lung* (wind): (mainly) light and coarse qualities
- *Tripa* (bile): (mainly) hot, oily, slightly malodorous qualities
- *Péken* (phlegm): (mainly) heavy, soft, static, oily, adhesive-sticky qualities

These factors coincide with the respective nature of the corresponding bodily energies. In addition to these effective qualities, there are the following **additional conditions:**
- For *Lung* (wind): in connection with heat
- For *Tripa* (bile): in connection with cold
- For *Péken* (phlegm): in connection with coolness

Conditions for manifestation:
  Lung (wind): cold
  Tripa (bile): heat
  Péken (phlegm): warmth (moisture)

Possibilities of pacification:
  Lung (wind): oily and warm
  Tripa (bile): blunt and cool
  Péken (phlegm): coarse, flexible, light, hot

These factors harmonize with the respective opposing factors of the corresponding bodily energy.

Entrances and Pathways for Diseases

To make it easier to understand the intrusion of illness and its spread within the body, the chapter on the entrances and pathways is placed before the explanation of the actual causes and conditions.

When the above-mentioned factors of the causes are activated by the corresponding conditions of manifestation, which are described in detail in the next chapter, the illness enters the body. At this time, the illness begins to spread in the skin, develops in the musculature, circulates in the vessels, settles into the bones, and then descends into the full organs. The illness ultimately concentrates in the hollow organs and settles there. This path of the spread of an illness is called the **entrance**. This path does not necessarily always take place in this order.

Each bodily energy has a specific *pathway*, meaning that diseases of the bodily energies circulate on these paths and can be recognized as such. In general, *Lung* (wind) primarily takes the path of the bones. *Tripa* (bile) primarily takes the path of the blood and sweat, and *Péken* (phlegm) moves in the rest of the bodily constituents.

The location of the pathways of Lung (wind):
- Middle to lower section of small intestine
- Bones (general)
- Hips (above all, hip joints)
- Joints (general)
- Skin
- Ears
- Large intestine (above all, during post-digestive phase)

The location of the pathways of Tripa (bile):
- Small intestine (navel area)
- Stomach
- Blood
- Sweat
- Lymph
- In the essence of the food
- Eyes
- Skin
- Between the digested and the undigested food (transition from stomach to small intestine)

The location of the pathways of Péken (phlegm):
- Chest
- Throat
- Lungs
- Head area
- In the essence of the food
- Musculature
- Fat

- Bone marrow
- Semen and ovum
- Feces
- Urine
- Nose
- Tongue
- Stomach

When complaints occur in the above-mentioned sections of the body, we can assume that there is an imbalance of the associated bodily energies.

General Symptoms of
Lung (Wind), Tripa (Bile), and Péken (Phlegm)

Each of the three bodily energies expresses itself in the related section of the body. Moreover, these energies can be specified for all of the corresponding symptoms. On this basis, we can more precisely distinguish which of the bodily energies is imbalanced.

General Symptoms of the Bodily Energy Lung
(Wind):

Since the bodily energy *Lung* is mainly located below the navel, most symptoms will also be manifested in this area. In addition, the following general symptoms are considered as typical for the *excess* or a disorder of the bodily energy *Lung*:
- Constant yawning and continuous sighing
- Frequently stretching
- Shivering, freezing, goose bumps, general sensation of coldness
- Astringent taste in mouth
- Body hurts during movement
- Indefinite pains (pain changes in intensity and quality, may sometimes be dull and then again shooting pain, etc.)
- Shifting pains (pain changes in location, may sometimes be in the area of the kidneys, then in the bones, in the joints etc.)

- General feeling of stiffness
- Hunger pain
- Rumbling in abdominal area
- Tendency toward constipation or diarrhea
- Tendency toward flatulence
- Impaired balance and feeling of dizziness
- Humming or ringing sound in the ears
- Feeling as if you had been hit with one-thousand sticks
- Feeling as if you had been tied up with ropes
- Feeling as if the skin and bones were separated from each other
- Feeling as if body parts were very taut (for example, the eyes)
- Impatience and general restlessness
- Dark skin color
- Sleeplessness
- Shooting pain beneath back of the head
- Shooting pain in nape of neck
- Shooting pain in cheekbones
- Shooting chest pain
- Pain in area of seventh cervical vertebra
- Coughing up foamy sputum in the morning
- Very talkative
- General touchiness and impatience
- Dry heaves(without vomiting)
- Weak memory (also general dullness of sensory organs)
- Mental instability (for example, moodiness)
- Pain after digestive phase (= about two hours after eating)
- Symptoms worsen about two hours after eating, at daybreak, and in the early evening
- Symptoms of the pulse and urine analysis (see *Pulse Diagnosis*, page 147f. and *Urine Diagnosis*, page 164f.)

If the symptoms of a *reduction* of the bodily energy *Lung* (wind) occur, these will mainly be expressed through the symptoms toward the bottom of the list describing an excess of *Péken* (phlegm). In addition, the following may occur:
- No desire to communicate
- Minimal energy, lethargy
- Physical discomfort

General Symptoms of the Bodily Energy Tripa
(Bile):

Since the bodily energy *Tripa* (bile) is mainly located between the diaphragm and the navel, most of the symptoms are also manifested in this area. In addition, the following symptoms are considered typical for an *excess* or a disorder of *Tripa*:

- Bitter taste in the mouth
- Sour taste in the mouth
- Drying of the nasal mucous membrane
- Vehement impulse to sleep during the day
- Sleeplessness, restless sleep
- Yellow coloration of stool and urine
- Yellow coloration of whites of eyes (sclera)
- Yellow coloration of skin
- Generally imprecise and slack movements
- Intense thirst
- General sensation of heat
- Tendency of profuse sweating
- Fever in the muscles
- Superficial fever
- Intense body odor
- General restlessness, ranging to aggressiveness
- Headache
- Pain during digestive phase (= about 1/2 to 2 hours after eating)
- Symptoms increase during digestive phase, around noon, and at midnight
- Symptoms of the pulse and urine analysis (see *Pulse Diagnosis,* page 147f. and *Urine Diagnosis,* page 164f.)

If the symptoms of a *reduction* of the bodily energy *Tripa* (bile) occur, these will mainly be expressed through:

- Dark skin color
- Loss of skin tone
- Loss of general body heat
- Sensation of coldness

General Symptoms of the Bodily Energy Péken
(Phlegm):

Since the bodily energy *Péken* (phlegm) is mainly located above the diaphragm, most of the symptoms are also manifested in this area. In addition, the following symptoms are considered typical for an *excess* or a disorder of the bodily energy *Péken*:

- Loss of appetite
- Swelling and/or pain directly after eating
- General sensation of fullness in the abdominal area
- Burping
- Tendency toward flatulence
- General weight gain
- General inflexibility of body and joints
- Diarrhea (contains undigested food remnants and/or phlegm)
- Weakening or loss of sense of taste
- Pale skin color
- Pale mouth area (tongue, gums, palate)
- Pale and swollen eyes
- Sluggish, feeble, and slack feeling of body and mind
- Constant sleepiness
- Difficulties in breathing
- Much mucus (stringy phlegm in the nose-throat area)
- Weak digestive heat
- Lethargy, hesitating, wavering
- Sensation of inner coldness
- Sensation of external coldness
- Symptoms worsen in damp weather
- Symptoms worsen directly after eating, mornings and evenings
- Symptoms of the pulse and urine analysis (see *Pulse Diagnosis,* page 147f. and *Urine Diagnosis,* page 164f.)

If the symptoms of a *reduction* of the bodily energy *Péken* (phlegm) occur, these will mainly be expressed through symptoms similar to those existing when there is an excess of *Lung* (wind) (racing heart, sensation of dizziness, etc.) and a general loosening of the joints.

On the basis of the symptoms of the three bodily energies listed above, you can classify many of the generally occurring complaints into one of these categories. Complex symptoms may naturally also develop as a result of an excess or disorder of more than one of the bodily energies. If you compare these with the tables at the end of the book to determine your personal basic constitution, as well as more intensively studying the chapters on seasonal changes, dietary habits, and behavior patterns—in addition to urine and pulse diagnosis—you can obtain a relatively precise picture of the inner correlations and imbalances of your own bodily energies.

Seasonal Changes

There are various divisions for the course of the Tibetan year. One factor that they all have in common is the division according to the course of the moon, meaning that the Tibetan year is a lunar year. In order to compensate for the missing number of days that occurs after several years, these days are lumped together into a leap month and added every three to four years. The actual calculation of the Tibetan New Year's celebration (Tib. *Losar*) is a science in itself, which is performed by the astrological staff of the Tibetan Medical & Astro Institute. The institute also publishes yearly calendars with the respective divisions. Here in the West, primarily the Tibetan calendar of *Rigpa*, the organization of Sogyal Rinpoche, can be mentioned in this respect. In the following section, the divisions are made according to the seasons of
- Spring
- Summer (the time of monsoon in the Tibetan calendar)
- Autumn
- Winter
- And a total of four phases in between the seasons.

The seasons—but not the phases in between—are then each divided into an early phase (= first half), as well as a late phase (= second half). Each season has a total of 72 days. Between each of the two main seasons, there are phases of 18 days each. This division can be translated to the seasonal cycles in Europe or North America. In this approach, the middle of the Tibetan spring corresponds to the Western beginning of spring and the middle of the Tibetan autumn corresponds to the Western beginning of autumn. The middle of the Tibetan summer corresponds to the Western summer solstice, and the middle of the Tibetan winter corresponds to the Western winter solstice.

Since a specific combination of elements predominates in each season and these in turn correspond with certain bodily energies, as well as dietary habits and behavior patterns, etc., it is easy to comprehend that certain elements—and therefore also the respective bodily energies—accumulate. This can lead to an excess and therefore an imbalance in the natural harmony of the body. (See *The Pulse of the Bodily Energies*, page 152f., about the distribution of the elements during the seasons and the chapter on distribution of the elements in behavior patterns and dietary habits, page 89f.)

As already described above, a disorder or imbalance of the bodily energies always occurs when the corresponding season is:
- Inadequate (for example, summer that is too cold)
- Excessive (for example, summer that is too hot)
- Unnatural (for example, no snow in winter).

Imbalances of the bodily energies can also occur because of the related dietary habits and behavior patterns. Examples of this excess may be dressing for winter in summer or constantly eating food that is too spicy. (For more details, see *Behavior and Dietary Habits*, page 89f.)

Times of Excessive Accumulation and Natural Pacification

We must differentiate between the times of (excessive) accumulation of a bodily energy, the manifestation period of a related illness, and the time of natural pacification of this bodily energy.

This subdivision can be also understood as the three phases of an overall process. During the *first phase*, there is an excessive accumulation of a bodily energy in its natural location. In addition, it is still disturbed by external factors. During this phase, the natural instinct of the body desires the contrary powers (for example, in the form of food).

During the *second phase*, the excessively accumulated bodily energy flows beyond its own location to the location of another bodily energy. During this time, the corresponding symptoms of the excessively accumulated and overflowing bodily energy become manifested.

During the *third phase*, the bodily energy finally returns to its own location. Now it has once again achieved its natural quantity and its natural location.

THE SEASONS OF ACCUMULATION FOR ONE BODILY ENERGY:

Lung (Wind):	In early summer
Tripa (Bile):	In summer and late summer
Péken (Phlegm):	In late winter

During each season, there are characteristically occurring illnesses (= time of activation or manifestation):

Lung (wind): *Lung* diseases primarily occur during the late summer and in autumn.

Tripa (bile): *Tripa* diseases primarily occur during (late summer and) autumn.

Péken (phlegm): *Péken* diseases primarily occur during (the late winter), spring, (and during the early summer).

THE SEASONS OF NATURAL PACIFICATION OF THE BODILY ENERGIES:

Lung (Wind):	Late autumn
Tripa (bile):	Early winter
Péken (phlegm):	Early summer

The Overall Picture Can Be Created
from the Above Factors:

The bodily energy *Lung* (wind) accumulates in the early summer through light and coarse seasonal conditions or dietary habits and behavior patterns. However, since these factors require the cold in order to manifest as a disease, they are kept in check by the warmth of the early summer. During late summer (Indian summer) or early autumn, this cold appears in the form of cold moisture in the morning and evening, as well as wind. The autumn has oily and warm active qualities in Tibetan medicine. As a result, it is possible that lesser imbalances of *Lung* balance themselves or that we can balance them by adding warm and oily active qualities to our dietary habits and behavior patterns.

The bodily energy **Tripa** (bile) accumulates during the late summer or early autumn through oily factors. However, these require warmth and even more oiliness to manifest themselves as imbalances or illness. This means that the cool and coarse factors of this season keep the manifestations in check. The *Tripa* disorders can only manifest themselves through the excessive oiliness of autumn. The coolness of early winter can compensate for lesser *Tripa* imbalances on its own, and the corresponding behavior patterns and dietary habits can support this process as well. The active quality of "blunt" can also be added to these.

The bodily energy *Péken* (phlegm) accumulates during the (late) winter through cool and heavy factors. However, these require warmth to manifest, which means that the cold of winter prevents this from happening. Only through the warmth of the spring sun can the *Péken* disorders then manifest themselves since the phlegm was too tough to overflow before then. The coarse and light conditions of the early summer calm lesser *Péken* disorders on their own. These may also be supported by the corresponding behavior patterns and dietary habits. The light, flexible, coarse, and hot active qualities can also be added here.

SUMMARY OF THE COURSE OF THE YEAR
IN THE NORTHERN HEMISPHERE

January/February	*Péken* (Phlegm)	accumulates
March/April	*Péken* (Phlegm)	rises
May/June	*Péken* (Phlegm)	diminishes
	Lung (Wind)	accumulates
July/August	*Lung* (Wind)	rises
	Tripa (Bile)	accumulates
September/Oktober	*Tripa* (Bile)	rises
	Lung (Wind)	diminishes
November/December	*Tripa* (Bile)	diminishes

Summary: The initial factors of the seasons, the sensory stimulation, and the dietary habits and behavior must either be inadequate, excessive, or inappropriate to produce a disorder or imbalance of the bodily energies.

THE THREE PHASES OF ACCUMULATION, ACTIVATION, AND PACIFICATION

Bodily Energy (through:)	1st Phase (= Collection) Factors with same active powers (such as diet)	2nd Phase (= Activation) Factors with same active powers (such as diet)	3rd Phase (= Pacification) Factors with opposing active powers (such as diet)
Lung	plus warm active powers	plus cold active powers	plus oily, warm etc.
Tripa	plus cool active powers	plus hot or warm active powers	plus heavy, cool etc.
Péken	plus cool active powers	plus warm active powers	plus coarse, light etc.

THE THREE BODILY ENERGIES IN RELATION TO THE SEASONAL CHANGES

Bodily Energy	Accumulation	Activation	Pacification
Lung	Early summer Autumn	Late summer	Late autumn
Tripa	Summer Late summer	Late summer Autumn	Early winter
Péken	Late winter	Spring (early summer)	Early summer

Energy Distribution During the Course of the Day

Even during a 24-hour cycle, there are natural shifts in the dynamic flow equilibrium of the elements:

Lung (Wind): Increase early evening (7-9 p.m.) and shortly before sunrise (3-5 a.m.)

Tripa (Bile): Increase around noon (11 a.m.- 1 p.m.), as well as around midnight (11 p.m.-1 a.m.)

Péken (Phlegm): Increase in the morning (9-11 a.m.) and evening (9-11 p.m.)

If a bodily energy is imbalanced, this will most likely be manifested at the corresponding time of day. Remedies also develop their strongest effects when they are taken at the corresponding times. Dietary habits and behaviors at the appropriate times can also more clearly develop their effects.

Examples:

1. People with a basic *Péken* constitution and/or a phlegm imbalance will, for example, have a hard time getting out of bed in the morning and also need quite a while to wake up. At this point in time, they should follow dietary habits and behavior patterns with opposing active powers. Instead of jam on bread and hot chocolate, breakfast should consist of a cup of hot water and something spicy. In addition, they should do physical exercises, at least in the morning.

2. Since the wind—and the bodily energy of *Lung*—sustains the mind, we can realize why the time between three and five a.m., which traditionally is selected quite often, is very advantageous for meditation. With the reverse logic, Tibetan medicine describes that too frequent or false meditation can lead to an excess of *Lung*. There are many other examples to show how necessary it is for each human being to live in natural harmony with the energy laws of the cosmos.

Non-Visible Forces:
"Demons" and
Biorhythmic-Planetary Influences

All of the phenomena that are called non-visible forces take place on a level that cannot be grasped by "normal" sensory reception. Only by contemplation with a pure heart and awake intelligence can we gain insight into these areas of being. The nature of cosmological medicine opens up in the synthesis between perception and scientific spirit. These phenomena range from diseases through planetary influences—such as infarcts, epilepsy, etc.—to infectious diseases like leprosy resulting from an injury of the spheres of specific types of spirit beings (such as *nagas*) or because of negative karmic factors. An illness based on karmic factors is frequently incurable and can solely be mitigated through rituals and the like. Occurrences related to "spirits" and "demons" express themselves in a clearly defined manner. Lamas can frequently exert a very positive influence on them.

Tibetan medicine has a differentiated system in this regard that is explained in various chapters of the third Medicine Tantra. For the more materially oriented Western individual, it is usually difficult to open up to these spheres of thought. It may help, for example, to imagine the possibility of emanations on the basis of water veins or faults. Electricity as a natural phenomenon or the sunspot rhythms, solar winds, etc. can be helpful in imagining these forces.

Another possibility within the scope of the psychological perspective could be mental suffering such as psychoses. Terry Clifford, in her book *The Diamond Healing*, writes: "The demons can very well be considered to be mental habits that become stronger and stronger—until the point in time that they assume a form...This can be compared to dreams. On the one hand, dreams are not real but while we dream them, they seem very realistic." "The demons can be understood as mental habits which become stronger and stronger until they take form—like our dreams. The dreams are not true, but they feel true when we are in them."

However, the Tibetan lamas also say that demons and spirit beings not only represent imaginary phenomenon but are also entities.

At least they exist in a form similar to everything else, which means dependent and not existing from within themselves. One of the major differences between the East and West in the fundamental way of viewing the universe becomes clear here. While the "natural science" of the West always assumes that matter has no life in it, for example, a Tibetan physician finds it quite obvious that all "things" have an essence of their own. One of the few exceptions in this regard in the Western tradition is the Spagyric-alchemical tradition and the anthroposophic medicine, which is partially related to the former.

Otherwise, "natural science" approaches tend toward seeing themselves as the only real, meaning comprehensible, criterion. This is why they categorize many of these phenomena as "unmeasurable in concrete terms" and therefore "unscientific." Things like viruses and bacteria obviously exist *despite* the recognition of non-visible phenomena. However, they may represent a possibility of an entity manifesting itself in the material sense—the weapon with which it fights, so to speak.

In any case, these entity manifestations—however we want to call them—represent a clear aspect of Tibetan medicine that should not be neglected. All cosmic-planetary factors have a distinct effect on the spheres and therefore also on the health of human beings. There is good reason why training in astrology is included in the medical education of a Tibetan physician. In the pharmacology of Tibetan medicine, each of the nine planets has specific substances ascribed to it. The nine planetary poisons (= the plants corresponding to the respective planets), as well as the toxic plants for the moon's nodes, are individually described in the Tibetan *materia medica*.

The planetary resonances constitute a clear factor of all dynamic life. Or, expressed in different terms: Every dynamic life process is basically a short-term "condensation" of the planetary resonances in connection with the personal resonance. (Strictly speaking, this differentiation is purely intellectual since "as above— so below," which occurs synchronistically.) Tibetan astrology is composed of—similar to the medicine—a mixture of Indian, Chinese, and the ancient Bon astrology. In addition, it has its own Buddhist-oriented character.

The main teachings about astrology came to Tibet with the Kalachakra Tantra around the year A.D. 1025. The Tibetan 60-year cycle based on it was systemized by the adept Atisha. Incidentally, *Kalachakra* means "wheel of time."

This is a highly complex Tantric teaching system of Tibetan spiritual training. It includes all of the instruction about elements in interaction with the cosmic phenomena, the corresponding dynamic relationships and temporal transformations, cosmology, all of the astrological calculations, the constellations of the solar system, etc., in a detailed manner.

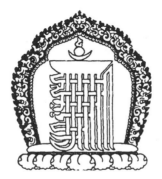

This portion is considered to be the "Outer Kalachakra." In the "Inner Kalachakra," all of these relationships are depicted within a human being. For this purpose, it uses a very clear system of the subtle body with all of its energy channels (sanskrit: *nadis*, tib.: *tsa)*, its energetic power wheels (sanskrit: *chakras*, tib.: *khorlo)*, the subtle winds (sanskrit: *prana*, tib.: *lung)*, as well as the essential energy drops (sanskrit: *bindu*, tib.: *thiglé*). The *Alternative Kalachakra* contains the teaching about the analogies between the Outer and the Inner Kalachakra.

All things of this universe are considered to be classified in a specific mandala. For example, our universe is within the order of a larger mandala. The earth, in turn, is found in the mandala of the planetary relationships. This order can naturally be seen in the surrounding world as well, from which the science of Tibetan geomancy is derived.

The human being as a representation of the universe on the small scale also forms a mandala in relation to his surrounding world, as well as in his personal body mandala, which is made of the above-described *nadis, chakras, thiglés*, etc. In the formation of the subtle and physical nerve channels during the first period of maturation in the womb, a specific mandala of consciousness is created. This is depicted in the adult human being as follows:

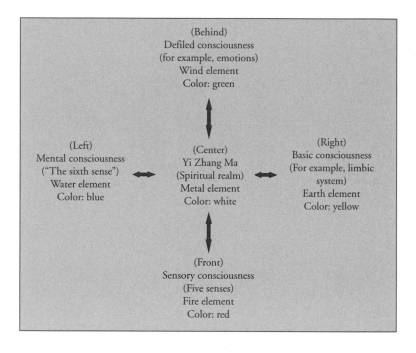

This "mandala" should not be understood in the anatomic sense. Instead, it reflects a stylized image of the various types of consciousness in a simplified form. So it can be viewed as an example of the universally occurring interlinking and fundamental order. The form of consciousness called *Yi Zhang Ma* is located in the heart and corresponds approximately to the spiritual, cosmic-loving sphere.

The basic consciousness corresponds in part with the personal (and, in an expanded form, the collective) unconscious. The defiled consciousness differentiates between the subject and the object, meaning the mental poisons of attachment, greed, anger, etc. act through this form of consciousness. The mental consciousness collects the impressions of the five senses and makes sure they are processed; in a certain sense, we could say it thinks. Here it is important to understand the Tibetan perspective, which says that human beings think with their hearts. The brain is solely the executing, meaning functional, organ. In Tibetan Buddhism, active compassion is part of the highest ideal.

Let us return to the topic of non-visible forces. These may be disturbed and then manifest themselves in a negative way such as in the form of an illness in the person who has caused this disruption. The Tibetan interpretation of the so-called *La* should be mentioned at this point. This *La* generally corresponds to the fundamental elemental life force of a human being.

A special form of taking the pulse is involved with the state of this "life force" and is done at the ulnary artery of the lower arm. Among other things, this fundamental life principle is responsible for the life force of a human being and moves through the body in the rhythmic cycles of the course of the moon. This monthly wandering movement of the *La* in the body can be used in meditation, for example, through the corresponding practices. The cycle corresponds with a moon cycle of somewhat more than 28 days. It begins on the sole of the foot (the right sole a man, the left for a woman) on the day of the new moon.

The *La* principle then wanders up to the crown on the respective side of the body. It reaches this point during the full moon, and then wanders down the other side of the body to the sole of the other foot. This results in a circular motion. However, this motion should not be understood as just linear since the *La* only stays in the head area for nine days, for example. (These days tend to be considered inauspicious for a visit to the dentist and the like. These are the days 5, 11, 12, 13, 15, 17, 20, 25, and 29, whereby the new moon is viewed as the 1st or 30th day.) A further practical application could be the use of foot reflexology massages and the like during the new moon phase.

Surgery, venesection, etc., should never take place on a part of the body where the *La* is situated at that moment since this vitality principle could suffer a lasting disruption as a result. This could definitely lead to a serious illness or even death. If you are interested in this principle in terms of European culture, read about Paracelsus' entity theory, which has certain similarities. The *La* can leave a person's body through the ring finger. These are occasions, for example, when people are "seen" somewhere other than where they actually are at the moment; or the respective person is in a coma or generally very weak condition.

The practices of black magic can also lastingly disrupt the *La*. Various practices, such as putting a red thread around the ring finger, are said to prevent this from occurring. (Incidentally, the *La* can return to the body despite the red thread being worn. This sheds a completely different light on the symbol of the wedding ring.) The *La* is not an independent entity, it is rather seen as the "presence" of the individual. This means that it tends to be equated with the basic elemental composition of a human being. So it also remains with the body after a person's death and dissolves into the elements in nine or thirteen years. If the *La* is disrupted at its location (meaning the cemetery), this can have negative effects on the person causing the disruption. The *La* also seems to be the principle that appears as a "ghost" of the deceased to the relatives.

Personal Signs of the Zodiac

Much of Tibetan astrology is involved with the elements. The astrological calculations have the objective of bringing the personal elemental distribution (such as the above-described *La*, the life force or so-called "wind horse," etc.) into a harmonious attunement with the planetary powers. Two separate calculation methods with different cycles (12-year cycle and 60-year cycle) are used, as well as one form of drawing the diagram.

However, the focus is meant to be on the relationship of the human being to the many different, non-visible levels and forces, all of which make a contribution to health and illness. Since it is understandably impossible to describe all of the individual aspects of the astrological calculations, etc. in this book, this chart provides simple assistance in calculating the auspicious and inauspicious days of the week. To do this, use the first table to find your personal sign of the zodiac. Then, with the help of the second table, you can select the appropriate days for activities, medical operations, etc.

Please note that the Tibetan New Year (=Losar) starts with one of the new moon phases between end of January and beginning of March.

TABLE OF THE PERSONAL SIGNS OF THE ZODIAC (60-YEAR CYCLE):

Fire/Hare	1867	1927	1987
Earth/Dragon	1868	1928	1988
Earth/Snake	1869	1929	1989
Metal/Horse	1870	1930	1990
Metal/Sheep	1871	1931	1991
Water/Monkey	1872	1932	1992
Water/Bird	1873	1933	1993
Wood/Dog	1874	1934	1994
Wood/Pig	1875	1935	1995
Fire/Rat	1876	1936	1996
Fire/Ox	1877	1937	1997
Earth/Tiger	1878	1938	1998
Earth/Hare	1879	1939	1999
Metal/Dragon	1880	1940	2000
Metal/Snake	1881	1941	2001
Water/Horse	1882	1942	2002
Water/Sheep	1883	1943	2003
Wood/Monkey	1884	1944	2004
Wood/Bird	1885	1945	2005
Fire/Dog	1886	1946	2006
Fire/Pig	1887	1947	2007
Earth/Rat	1888	1948	2008
Earth/Ox	1889	1949	2009
Metal/Tiger	1890	1950	2010

Metal/Hare	1891	1951	2011
Water/Dragon	1892	1952	2012
Water/Snake	1893	1953	2013
Wood/Horse	1894	1954	2014
Wood/Sheep	1895	1955	2015
Fire/Monkey	1896	1956	2016
Fire/Bird	1897	1957	2017
Earth/Dog	1898	1958	2018
Earth/Pig	1899	1959	2019
Metal/Rat	1900	1960	2020
Metal/Ox	1901	1961	2021
Water/Tiger	1902	1962	2022
Water/Hare	1903	1963	2023
Wood/Dragon	1904	1964	2024
Wood/Snake	1905	1965	2025
Fire/Horse	1906	1966	2026
Fire/Sheep	1907	1967	2027
Earth/Monkey	1908	1968	2028
Earth/Bird	1909	1969	2029
Metal/Dog	1910	1970	2030
Metal/Pig	1911	1971	2031
Water/Rat	1912	1972	2032
Water/Ox	1913	1973	2033
Wood/Tiger	1914	1974	2034
Wood/Hare	1915	1975	2035
Fire/Dragon	1916	1976	2036
Fire/Snake	1917	1977	2037
Earth/Horse	1918	1978	2038
Earth/Sheep	1919	1979	2039
Metal/Monkey	1920	1980	2040
Metal/Bird	1921	1981	2041
Water/Dog	1922	1982	2042
Water/Pig	1923	1983	2043
Wood/Rat	1924	1984	2044
Wood/Ox	1925	1985	2045
Fire/Tiger	1926	1986	2046

You can determine your personal Tibetan sign of the zodiac in connection with your personal element through this overview. To find the auspicious and inauspicious days of the week, you only need your personal sign of the zodiac.

On the basis of the auspicious days of the week you can, for example, discover which day is fundamentally better for starting a new project, etc. For the Tibetan medicine, it is important to know the best-possible time for diagnosis and/or treatment. This "best" day is naturally the one on which your personal energies are in the most harmonious attunement with the cosmic energies. In addition to several other finer factors—like the individual rhythm, the course of the moon, etc.—the following table can also be used for this purpose.

Zodiac sign	Auspicious day	Inauspicious day
Rat	Tuesday	Saturday
Ox	Wednesday	Thursday
Hare + Tiger	Saturday	Friday
Dragon	Wednesday	Thursday
Snake + Horse	Friday	Wednesday
Sheep	Montag	Thursday
Bird + Monkey	Thursday	Tuesday
Dog	Wednesday	Thursday
Pig	Tuesday	Saturday

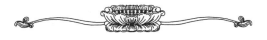

Section III

Behavior and Dietary Patterns

General Behavior Patterns

Physical, emotional, as well as mental behavior patterns that are practiced in an inadequate, excessive, or distorted manner can create the conditions for manifestation, meaning the immediate causes of an illness. The distinguished culture of the Tibetan people has developed very clear ethics and many of the general rules for behavior in Tibetan medicine are primarily related to irreproachable behavior in everyday life. The purpose of these rules is to avoid anger and strife, and therefore also the negative effects that this has on body and mind.

Once we recognize that every negative action results in negative consequences for the person who has taken it, then these guidelines are actually quite clear and easy to understand. These specific recommendations are not meant to cause us to monitoring ourselves in an overly rigid manner. Instead, they can very fundamentally help us to perceive our own structures and the effects that these have on our general condition. They are not meant to restrict us in our individual spontaneity. Some aspects should also be understood in relation to the culturally specific Tibetan background.

Some of the very general recommendations include keeping our word of honor, not letting others prevent us from engaging in honorable activities, and not becoming involved in strife and quarrelsome talk. We should behave in an honest and respectful manner toward our relatives and those who are entrusted to us (which also includes "subordinates"). Those who are our superiors should not be viewed with envy.

The recommendations that we should not expose ourselves to unbridled sensory experiences or spend time in places where killing takes place (like slaughterhouses) or where there are bandits ("bandits" can be understood here both in the literal sense and the figurative sense as unpleasant people) also tend to be general in nature.

In addition, they advise against such actions as adultery or sexual intercourse with a pregnant woman or a woman during menstruation. The latter should not be understood as patriarchal thinking but has a medical reason: menstrual blood also contains physical "impurities." For a man, this could lead to illness. For a woman, the result could be congestion in the flow of the blood, which could lead to *Lung* disorders.

In Buddhism, all sentient beings are considered from the perspective of possible liberation from suffering since every being would like to be happy. Consequently, the ideals of a spiritual mental attitude are depicted within the context of the behavior patterns. Above all, this means a free manner of giving and compassion toward all beings suffering from misery, sadness, poverty, illness, etc. From the Buddhist perspective, we should refrain from the ten negative actions of the body, the speech, and the mind. Among others, these include killing, stealing, lying, malice, desire, false attitudes, as well as vain and divisive chatter. It is important for every human being to be able to be friendly and happy and to develop a basic attitude of spiritual expansiveness.

Triggering Conditions for an Excess of Lung, Tripa, and Péken

Triggers for an Excess of Lung

General: Light and coarse conditions such as
- Talking for a long time (above all, with an empty stomach)
- Worry, sorrow, and crying
- Too little sleep or interrupted or light sleep
- Exhaustion (above all, through mental exertion)
- Too many sensory impressions (such as sitting too long in front of the computer or television, constantly listening to music, etc.)
- Fasting or eating on an irregular basis
- Increasing age (starting around the mid-fifties)
- Distorted sensory perceptions (for example, because of horror films)
- Fear, shocking experiences
- Suppression of physical expression (for example, sneezing, yawning, panting, and holding back the intestinal gas or the urge to urinate or have a bowel movement)

- Drafty, windy, cold, high-lying regions
- Looking down from great heights
- Wide waters
- Light, cool, and coarse diet (for example, coffee, tea, pork; see *Dietary Habits,* page 98f.)
- Seasonal conditions (see next chapter)

Trigger for an Excess of Tripa (Bile)

General: sharp and hot conditions such as

- Physical exertion
- Middle period of life (about 15-65)
- Too much sunbathing
- Consumption of alcohol
- Hot, dry areas
- Sharp, hot, oily, and sour diet (see *Dietary Habits,* page 98f.)
- Places where a high aggression potential prevails
- Seasonal conditions (see next chapter)

Trigger for an Excess of Péken (Phlegm)

General: Heavy and oily conditions such as

- Too much sleep or sleeping during the day
- Laying or sitting on damp group (for example, in a meadow)
- Childhood (up to about 15 years of age)
- Heavy, oily, and sweet diet (see *Dietary Habits,* page 98f.)
- Eating too much and too often
- Damp regions
- Too little physical exercise
- Seasonal conditions (see next chapter)
- Suppression of bodily needs (for example, nose blowing or spitting)

Seasonal Behavior

Since every human being has an individual distribution of the bodily energies or elements, it is necessary to adapt personal dietary habits and behavior patterns in keeping with the dynamic processes of the elements during the course of the year. You should basically keep in mind that the energies of the sun—and therefore the elements of fire and air with their qualities coarse, hot, and sharp, etc.—continuously increase from the time of the winter solstice until the time of summer solstice. In this process, the accumulated energy of the body is used by the elements of wind and fire; we could also speak of burning in this context.

From the time of the summer solstice to the winter solstice, the energy of the moon—and therefore the elements water and earth with their qualities heavy, solid, sweet, etc.—increases. During this time period, energy is basically gathered. In Tibetan medicine, the time of the winter solstice is considered to be the greatest accumulation of energy; the time around the summer solstice is viewed as the time with the lowest energy reserves.

The recommendations regarding sexual life result from this perspective. While there are no restrictions in terms of the frequency of sexual contact during the winter, a maximum of once every two weeks is advisable during the summer. The recommendation for spring and autumn is engaging in sexual intercourse every two days at most.

Since the Western individual is usually physically active during the summer and engages in sports, this recommendation may not be easy for the Western mind to understand. To do so, we must take a closer look at the relationship between the prevailing and the substance-giving elements. While the highest level of energy and power (fire and wind) prevails during the summer, the body's substance energy is at its lowest level (water and earth).

But the sexual desire correlates with fire and air, meaning the energy that prevails in the outside world at this time. If this fire is excessively fanned, there will be an even greater loss of the substance-giving elements of water and earth. This would lead to a reduction of the bodily constituents and ultimately to the exhaustion of the bodily energies.

Another reason for this recommendation can be found in the fact that the body doesn't receive enough cooling in the summer, which leads to overheating. The desire for sexual activity that may occur more intensely during the summer should therefore not be confused with the inner energy relationships. Exactly the opposite conditions prevail during the winter, creating a type of "reciprocity." The natural outside world gathers itself and the substance-forming elements in the body accumulate as well. Now that this substance is abundantly available, it can also be used. You can imagine the ratio between the two forces like a loop running in opposite directions.

Spring

The time for the recommended dietary habits and behavior patterns during the spring (from March/April to mid-May) begins six weeks before the spring equinox on March 21st and ends six weeks later. During the winter, the bodily energy *Péken* accumulates. But, because of the existing cold, it stays viscous in the body. Through the warmth of the sun during the above-specified time from mid-February to the end of April, *Péken* begins to dissolve and "melts." As a result, this accumulated *Péken* energy could smother the digestive heat, which is why it needs additional support. *Péken* also stimulates the occurrence of the corresponding "phlegm" dissease.

This effect can be counteracted with sharp, hot, bitter, and astringent qualities. Examples of foods with these qualities are all dishes with spicy seasoning, onions, cress, lamb, mutton, cooked grains, ginger (for example, as a decoction), and honey. A glass of hot water also supports the digestive heat during this period. Lemon juice can be added to the hot water to dissolve the excess phlegm. Examples of behavior with these qualities are light exercise several times a day, walking, and jogging.

After the barren winter, this is also the time to please your senses with sweet-scented fragrances and Mother Nature's newly grown green. In addition, the excess *Péken* that has accumulated in the skin during the winter can be removed through "peeling" treatments on a regular basis. A powder made of dried lentils or peas is traditionally used in Tibet for this purpose. After vigorously rubbing it into the skin, wash the powder off again with soap.

Early Summer and Summer

This season is followed by the transitional period of early summer (mid-May to mid-June), during which somewhat cool and sweet foods are recommended. This period transitions relatively easily into the hot mid-summer months. The dietary habits and behavior patterns during the summer (mid-June to mid-August) are primarily derived from the heat and the insolation. Because of these aspects, the oily factors of the moon that were accumulated during the winter are burned and the body increasingly loses its power. Avoid all foods that are salty, sour, or hot and counteract the burning process with the factors sweet, oily, cool, and light in a natural form.

Foods with these qualities are all fruits (except for citrus fruits), potatoes, saffron, rice (as porridge or roasted), barley, wheat, meat broth, noodles, artichokes, legumes like peas and beans, milk, butter, fish, game, beef, pork, and so forth. If you drink alcohol, you should mix it with water during this season.

In terms of the behavior patterns required for the summer, it is advisable not to exhaust yourself too much. Don't spend too much time in the (direct) sunshine, wear light and thin clothing, and bathe in cool water instead of hot water. Sit in the shade of fragrant trees and enjoy the gentle breeze of the wind. Create an aromatic, cool atmosphere in your house by keeping the shutters closed and displaying flowers or spraying a mixture of water and essential essences with an atomizer.

Late Summer and Early Autumn

In late summer and early autumn (end of August to mid-September), the cooler and damper qualities appear through the morning dew and the rain, as well as the winds that arise. This weakens the digestive heat, which must be strengthened through the compensating dietary habits and behaviors. To do this, it is often necessary to produce additional heat, which means that the qualities of sweet, sour, salty, light, warm, and oily must be strengthened. The corresponding foods for this purpose are meat soup, sesame oil, clarified butter, (fatty) mutton and lamb, chicken, rabbit, fish, roasted oats, corn, rye, lentils, potatoes, grapes, garlic, nutmeg, and coriander. In terms of behavior recommendations, the most important one is to avoid cool places.

Autumn

Autumn (mid-September to the end of October) has warm and oily qualities in the Tibetan perspective. As a result of the food in late summer and early autumn, and these qualities, the bodily energy Tripa (bile) can rise. A diet with sweet, bitter, and astringent qualities will prevent this occurrence and dissolve the bodily energy of bile. Examples of foods with these qualities are artichokes, fenugreek, buckwheat, corn, fish, legumes (above all, lentils), apricots, plums, mangos, and so forth. The recommendations regarding behavior are mainly related to the home environment. You can either spray a mixture of water with white sandalwood and camphor or burn the same mixture as incense in order to enjoy a pleasant smell in the house.

Winter

Above all, *the early winter* (November/December) brings with it the factor of cold. The skin pores contract. Together with the fire-accompanying wind (*Lung*), this makes the digestive heat very intense. In order to prevent the digestive heat from consuming the bodily constituents, you should eat a great deal during this season. This gives the digestive heat the "substance" that it can work on.

The food should have the qualities of sweet, sour, and salty. The ingested food can be fat and oily, such as fatty mutton, chicken, fish, clarified butter, meat soup, and so forth. In terms of behavior, it is advisable to rub your body with sesame oil (or another type of warming seed oil) after bathing, sit in front of a fire or in the sun without overheating yourself. You should generally wear warm clothing and occasionally use a warm compress, if necessary.

In late winter (January/February), *Péken* gathers in the abdomen, which in turn is influenced by the dietary habits and behavior patterns described in the paragraph on "Spring.".

Summary

The diet should be:

• Bitter, hot, and astringent with coarse active powers in *spring*. The digestive heat should be strengthened.

• Sweet and cool in the *early summer*.

• Sweet, oily, cool, and light in *mid-summer*. Be sure to avoid the tastes sour, hot, and salty.

• Sweet, sour, light, warm, and oily in *late summer* and *early autumn*. The digestive heat should be supported.

• Sweet, bitter, and astringent in *autumn*.

• Sweet, sour, and salty in *early winter*. Be sure you have enough substance for the digestive heat.

• *In late winter*: Transition to the diet described under "Spring."

Dietary Habits

General Advice and Recommendations

The food and drink that we consume every day can be used in a distinctly sensible and tasty way to maintain the body's inner balance of the elements. High-quality food from organic cultivation should be preferred over a diet that is only "rich" in quantity. Whether food comes from organic cultivation and therefore also does justice to its purpose as a life-supporting substance is not only evident just in terms of the taste. In the long run, it also makes a difference whether it fulfills its purpose as living food—filled with life and necessary for life—or whether it just meets the requirements of a "filler." Locally grown products should generally be preferred because the body is better adapted to their corresponding environmental conditions than those of exotic products.

Poor digestive heat based on years of improper eating, meaning a diet not in harmony with the individual bodily energies, causes many illnesses in the Western industrial nations. Additional dietary mistakes that can be observed are deficiency symptoms because of excessive consumption of sugar and animal products. Tibetan medicine does not at all reject eating animal products like meat, eggs, butter, etc. For certain deficiency conditions, these foods can have distinct life-supporting properties. How you act in terms of these products is naturally a personal matter that should also be decided with respect to your type of constitution.

The success of every therapeutic effort is only possible when we simultaneously coordinate the diet with individual bodily energy distribution, meaning the basic constitution. We could even go so far as to claim that without adhering to the corresponding dietary rules it is practically impossible to maintain good health or become healthy.

The question of diet is a fundamental topic for every individual. It should be considered without prejudices and dogmas. The classically prescribed dietary rules in Tibetan medicine are based on the living conditions of a people who mainly live in a cold and windy climate above 4000 meters. Consequently, these rules must be adapted to the prevalent living conditions and climate outside of Tibet. On the basis of the ingenious system of linking the taste and the elements, this is possible in a universal manner for every individual under all of the prevailing living conditions.

A gathering of one of the bodily energies always takes place when its characteristic quality is strengthened. In the case of the diet, this gathering process takes place through the ingestion of foods with the same basic qualities as the corresponding bodily energies. The composition of the elements in the foods is determined on the basis of the six tastes.

The treatises of the Medicine Buddha offer the following *basic rules regarding the diet:*

1. Do not eat old food.
These foods have the tendency of developing a "heavy" active power, which can lead to disorders of the digestive heat. In addition, old foods tend to be a breeding ground for all types of bacteria, mold, etc. Food kept in the refrigerator also becomes "heavy" in the course of time and should be used as quickly as possible. (Heat first!)

2. Avoid constantly eating acidic foods.
These include sour pickles, "mixed pickles," and basically everything that has been pickled. When eaten excessively, food with the taste of "sour" (and "hot") attack the seven bodily constituents, among other things, and lead to illness as a result. Above all, people with skin problems should first remove all acidic foods from their diet!

3. Avoid excessive consumption of raw, green leafy vegetables.
This advice is mainly meant for people with weakened digestive energy and is not related to teachings about vitamins. The structure of leafed vegetables, such as lettuce, is very difficult to break down. Moreover, the elements of earth and water are intensified when we eat raw vegetables or lettuce. Earth and water form the basis for the bodily energy *Péken* (phlegm), and *Péken* in turn leads to suppression of the digestive heat.

So if you have weakened digestive powers, avoid everything raw (above all, raw leafy vegetables) until the digestive heat has been restored. If you would like to eat raw lettuce, etc., then do so before the main meal, if possible. Totally avoid having a light salad as dinner since this cannot be completely digested and will cause fermentation in the intestine. This fermentation process leads to straining the entire metabolic system, especially the liver. There have frequently been cases showing that people who only eat raw foods will eventually suffer from serious liver disorders.

The personal physician to the Dalai Lama, Dr. Tenzin Choedrak, points out that an excessive consumption of raw foods leads to an increase in the bodily energy of *Péken*. This, in turn, can cause an increase in the fat content of the blood (hyperlipoidemia), that can lead to diseases of the heart, etc.

Additional General Advice in Relation to Diet

- Should a slight imbalance of a bodily energy prevail, *fasting* is a simple and very good remedy to begin with. However, you should not overdo fasting since it can cause an excess of the bodily energy *Lung* (wind). People with a strong constitution usually have no problem when they eat nothing for up to three days, but they should be very careful to consume enough fluids during this time period. However, people who are somewhat weaker or dominated by *Lung* (wind) should initially "fast" by just consuming a rice broth or a meat broth for one day. This will generally relieve the metabolism without weakening the body too much.
- Be sure to always drink *adequate liquids*. It is best to do this in the form of clear water or a suitable herb tea. You can either create the herb teas yourself according to your constitution type or purchase tea mixtures made according to Tibetan recipes. "Adequate liquids" is naturally a relative statement since you must adapt it to your constitution type, your age, and your behavior patterns. A person with a *Tripa* basic constitution at a medium age and with intense physical strain in great heat represents the extreme case here. He will probably have a hard time just keeping up with how much cooling liquid he should be drinking...On the other hand, a very young person with a *Péken* basic constitution and little exercise in cold climatic conditions represents the other extreme. He should naturally drink liquids ranging from warm to hot and also will require much less fluid than the first case. Liquids are basical-

ly indispensable for the identification of tastes, as well as for the digestive process. In addition, they also satisfy the bodily constituents. An adequate amount of liquid also facilitates easier detoxification of the tissue and a good bowel movement. Remember that human beings consist of up to 75% water! Through respiration and the skin alone, about three-quarter quarts of liquid are converted in the course of 24 hours.

- *Do not drink any cold beverages before, during, or after the meal.* This will only lead to an unnecessary strain on the digestive heat—unless it is overly active. Eating ice cream as dessert should be an absolute exception, especially for people with a *Péken* or *Lung* constitution.

- You should usually drink *most of the liquid* (during and) *after the meal.*

- *Chew very thoroughly*—at best until the food is in an almost fluid state. This act of chewing leads to an increase in the "mixing phlegm." Since the food is already separated in the mouth, this will relieve the digestive heat. Above all, people with weak digestive heat should heed this advice.

- A *basic rule of the teaching of Tibetan medicine* says that half of the food eaten should consist of solid substance. One-fourth should be liquid, and the remaining quarter of the stomach should stay empty.

- *Don't eat any further meals until the previously eaten food has been completely digested.* This strains the digestive heat and the organs, among other things, in an unnecessary manner and creates disorders of the bodily energy *Lung* (wind).

- *Don't eat your food too hot*—lukewarm is better. In winter you need more heat in the form of warm food than in summer.

- *Avoid unripe food.* (Fruit, vegetables, and grain that is still "green")

- *Eating on a regular basis* is an important component of a healthy diet. The main warm meal should be eaten at noon.

- Bring *a sense of tranquility* into the way that you eat. Leave yourself enough time to eat and avoid thinking, talking, or reading about unpleasant or burdensome things. Also avoid subjecting yourself to these types of programs on the radio or television. Emotional and mental impulses during the meal also have an effect on the three bodily energies.

Advice Related
to Digestive Heat

As already discussed in the chapter on *Digestive Heat* (see page 50f.), this digestive fire or "fire of life" represents an essential basic component for the health and well-being of every human being.

In a person with very active or excessive digestive heat (*Tripa* disorders and/or *Tripa* basic constitution), the digestive fire burns the bodily constituents. In the long run, this consumes the body and represents serious injury to the state of health. People in this condition must absolutely be examined by a practitioner skilled in naturopathy!

As an additional(!) self-help measure, all of the dietary habits and behavior patterns can be employed that oppose the bodily energy *Tripa* (bile). If you are in this situation, frequently drink cool water and do not eat anything spicy, for example. Caution: Do not additionally also stimulate the bodily energy *Lung* (wind)—because wind fans the fire! Food and/or medications with bitter and tart, astringent active powers may possibly provide relief, but they should only be used in moderate amounts.

However, the digestive fire is too weak for most people. Even if they frequently look well fed: according to the Tibetan perspective, this state represents a condition of "mock health." Because of the insufficient division of the ingested food, which results in a less than optimally functioning formation of the bodily constituents, the undigested portions are deposited directly into the fatty tissue. The manifestation of an illness is therefore just a matter of time respectively of the triggering conditions.

The following advice is related to activating the digestive heat. When reading it, please be absolutely aware that only the proper proportion in harmony with the individually prevailing basic constitution, together with healthy common sense, can lead to lasting success. One example of this principle is eating mutton, which can lead to problems with the bodily energy *Lung* (wind) when too much of it is consumed. The excessive consumption of ginger can lead to an imbalance of the bodily energy *Tripa* (bile). So the amount determines whether a substance is a poison or a healing remedy.

Advice for Maintaining and Activating the Digestive Heat:

- Mainly eat foods with the active powers of "light" and "warm" (cf. the chapter *The Active Powers of the Types of Taste,* page 119f.)
- The pomegranate (especially the seeds) is considered an outstanding plant for activating the digestive heat.
- Drinking hot water is a time-tested, simple measure; it's best to do this before, during, and after meals.
- Boiling some ginger for about ten minutes is very beneficial for the digestive heat. This drink should be consumed as hot as possible. You can recognize whether you have exceeded the proper dosage if the stool becomes too soft.
- Honey intensifies the digestive heat and can be mixed in with the ginger decocion, for example.
- Garlic
- Onions
- (Black) radish
- Red radish
- Fish (also very good for the stomach)
- Mutton or lamb
- Smoking suppresses the digestive heat to a large extent.
- A hot salt compress on the liver area (= beneath the right costal arch)
- Eating something slightly acidic before the meal increases the digestive heat
- Drinking a digestion tea is very beneficial. (See *Adresses,* on page 240.)
- Avoid all foods with the same active powers and principles as the bodily energy *Péken* (phlegm).
- Observe the advice on digestive heat regarding how to eat during the course of the seasons that is found in the chapter on *Seasonal Behavior* (see page 93f.)

Fundamental Nutritional Instructions for the Constitutional Types

This information is meant for the case of a corresponding basic constitution and/or an excess of one of the three bodily energies.

Lung (wind)

- Be absolutely sure to take enough time to eat and keep the atmosphere tranquil
- Have regular eating habits
- Be sure not to let your stomach get completely empty
- Several smaller meals are more beneficial than one overly abundant meal
- Warm soup (including meat soup) is also very beneficial
- A small, sweet dessert provides a sense of well-being
- Drinks should always be at least room temperature
- Avoid cold foods (ice cream and the like) and cold beverages
- Cooked foods should be clearly preferred over raw foods
- Avoid coffee
- Don't drink too much black tea (drink only with plenty of milk!)
- Don't eat pork
- Avoid the taste of "sour" (vinegar, pickled foods, olives, etc.)
- Don't eat food that's too spicy (see *Types of Tastes* under "hot," on page 113f.)
- You can drink a glass of wine or beer with your meal (afterward is even better), but no hard liquor!

Tripa (bile)

- Allow yourself a calm atmosphere while eating.
- Drink cool drinks (water, if possible) during meals.
- You can eat raw foods because of your high level of digestive heat
- Avoid fat and oily foods (fried foods, sauces, etc.)
- Drink very little alcohol in general, especially no strong hard liquor
- A cool, sweet dessert (like fruit salad) is beneficial
- Avoid hot spices, ginger, mustard, and horseradish
- Avoid radishes and hot peppers
- Avoid olives
- Avoid vinegar (see *Types of Tastes* under "sour," on page 111).
- Eat very few eggs
- Avoid sesame (for example, on bread or as oil)
- Don't eat any soya products (such as miso)

- Avoid yeast products
- Don't eat your food too hot
- Basically avoid coffee

Péken (Phlegm)

- Drink warm to hot water before and after meals
- Don't drink too much in general; instead, emphasize solid foods.
- Steamed vegetables are ideal
- Avoid all heavy, fat, and oily foods (fried foods, sauces, etc.)
- Avoid cabbage, cauliflower, and the like.
- Don't eat too many carrots or bell peppers
- Drink very little alcohol (especially beer)—if you do, then a little glass of hard liquor after the meal
- Reduce your consumption of sweets as much as possible
- Don't eat very much at once and don't eat too frequently
- Observe the recommendations regarding the activation of the digestive heat.

The Types of Tastes

We mainly experience the Types of Tastes (Tib. *ro*) through the tongue and the palate. All types of tastes possess a respective elemental composition (and therefore also active power = healing power). As a result, they present an ideal medium for identifying the composition of the elements in plants, foods, etc.

THE SIX TYPES OF TASTES ARE:

- Sweet   (tib. *gnarwa*)
- Sour   (tib. *kyurwa*)
- Salty   (tib. *lentsawa*)
- Bitter   (tib. *khawa*)
- Hot   (tib. *tsawa*)
- Astringent   (tib. *kawa*)
  (tart, biting)

The above order of the types of tastes reflects the descending active power of a remedy. This means that a sweet remedy is stronger in its effect than a sour remedy. Sour is stronger in its effect than salty, and salty is stronger in its effect than bitter, etc.

These six types of tastes can be divided into an even finer differentiation by mutually combining them. This results in the following classifications for the taste of "sweet": the sweet of sweet, the sour of sweet, the salty of sweet, the bitter of sweet, the hot of sweet, and the astringent of sweet. The same types of classifications can also be done for the other tastes.

ALL SIX TYPES OF TASTES HAVE CHARACTERISTIC QUALITIES THAT ALLOW US TO RECOGNIZE THEM:

- The *sweet* taste sticks to the tongue, is tasty, and creates a desire for it.

- The *sour* taste causes people to make a face. It also produces saliva.

- The taste of *salty* also provides increased salivation and has an additional heating effect.

- *Bitter* improves the mouth odor, is considered an appetite depressant, and a regulative for the digestion.

- Hot produces a flow of tears, burns on the tongue and palate, and has a strong heating effect.

- An astringent (= tart) taste sticks to the palate and creates a roughened feeling. It is also classified with the active power of "coarse."

The tastes have both a quantitative and a qualitative aspect. This means that a substance will show the respective elements (quantitative aspect), as well as activating the corresponding elements in the body by means of the energetic interlinking (= qualitative or energetic aspect).

For example, the bitter taste is certain to result in the activation of the digestive glands. This makes it clear that not only the substance is effective as a healing remedy but the taste in itself. The fact of energetic activation through the taste is very important for understanding the Tibetan teachings about nutrition and the compounding of medicines.

If a person has a healthy instinct, as well as healthy common sense, then he will primarily select foods that serve the sustenance or balancing of his bodily energies. So health can also be very tasty!

The Types of Tastes in Relation
to the Elements

All things in the universe are made of the five elements. The element earth is responsible for the basis or the foundation. The moisture is added by the element water. The element fire provides the necessary heat, and the element wind (air) is responsible for movement. The fifth element—space—pervades the other four elements and makes available the required space for the development of the activities.

The formation of the tastes through the elements takes place in the following manner:

FORMATION OF THE TYPES OF TASTES
THROUGH THE ELEMENTS

Type of taste. . . . . Elements

Sweet . . . . Earth + Water
Sour . . . . Earth + Feuer
Salty . . . . Fire + Water
Bitter . . . . Water + Wind
Hot . . . . Fire + Wind
Astringent (tart) . . . . Earth + Wind

Every Element Has Characteristic Qualities or Active Powers:

The element *earth* has the characteristic active powers heavy, solid, blunt, smooth, oily (greasy-fatty), and dry. The task of the element earth is developing, forming, and solidifying the body. Earth cures diseases of the bodily energy *Lung* (wind).

The element *water* has the characteristic active powers liquid, cool, heavy, blunt, oily, as well as supple (or pliable). The tasks of the element water are making moisture available and solidifying the body or keeping it flexible. Water cures diseases of the bodily energy *Tripa* (bile).

The element *fire* has the characteristic active powers hot, sharp, coarse, light, and oily, as well as flexible. Fire is responsible for the thermodynamics of the body, as well as ripening the bodily constituents. Furthermore, fire provides a clear complexion and healthy skin. Fire cures diseases of the bodily energy *Péken* (phlegm).

The element *wind* (air) has the characteristic active powers light, flexible, cold, coarse, absorbing, and dry. Above all, wind has the task of organizing the body, as well as distributing nutriments and waste materials. Wind cures diseases of the bodily energies *Péken* (phlegm) and *Tripa* (bile).

The element *space* has no characteristic qualities. It pervades all the other elements and gives them the possibility of developing. Space has the task of making "space" available. Space cures diseases of all three bodily energies, as well as combinations of them.

The following statement is written at the end of the corresponding passage of the classic text: "Through the depiction of the elements and their combinations, it becomes clear that... whether it is natural or has been incorporated into a compound, there is nothing on the surface of the earth that is not a medicine." In his introduction to the translation of the *Quintessence Tantras*, Dr. Barry Clark tells the story that took place during Buddha's lifetime:

Jivaka, Buddha's famous personal physician, asked his disciples to go out and bring him substances that were not medicine. By the end of the first day, all of the disciples—except one—had returned. Only after several days did the last disciple come back, covered with dust. He told Jivaka that he unfortunately could find nothing at all that could not be used as a medicine. This was the answer for which Jivaka had waited...

All substances (healing remedies, foods, etc.) with an upward directed tendency are formed by the rising forces of the elements fire and air. All substances with a downward directed tendency are formed by the descending forces of the elements of water and earth.

Functions of the Tastes and Their Natural Occurrence

1. The Sweet Taste

- Has a regenerating effect
- Increases body strength
- Increases the bodily constituents
- Promotes longevity
- Helps in development of the body
- Helpful in maintaining the body
- Beneficial for growth of hair
- Beneficial for clarity of sensory organs
- Cures poisoning
- Cures hoarseness and other throat diseases
- Cures diseases of the lungs
- Cures diseases of the bodily energies *Lung* (wind) and *Tripa* (bile)
- Cures diseases of combined *Lung-Tripa* imbalances
- Beneficial for children
- Beneficial for older people
- Beneficial for people suffering from undernourishment

Excessive intake:
- Increases the bodily energy *Péken* (phlegm)
- Increases fatty tissue
- Reduces digestive heat
- Can lead to excessive growth of the glands (thyroid gland, pancreas)
- Increases need for sleep
- Increases mental sluggishness

Naturally occurs in:
- Basically all natural substances containing sugar or starch
- (Almost) all types of grain
- Linseed
- Sesame
- Vegetable oils

- Nuts, almonds, etc.
- Dates, figs, ripe grapes, and many other fruits
- Saffron
- Licorice
- Raisins
- Honey
- Molasses
- Sweet potatoes
- (Hokkaido) pumpkin
- Carrots
- (Almost) all types of meat (please observe special rule related to therapeutic effectiveness!)
- Milk products

2. The Sour Taste

- Increases bodily heat
- Improves the appetite
- Helps decomposition of food (= digestant)
- Causes loss of sensitivity (= slightly pain-relieving when applied externally)
- Sets the blocked bodily energy *Lung* (wind) back into motion (when applied externally)
- Has invigorating effect
- Helps clear senses
- Beneficial against *Lung* diseases
- Beneficial against *Péken* diseases

Excessive intake:
- Increases the bodily energy *Tripa* (bile)
- Excessively increases the blood
- Allows the body to become limp and wilted
- Creates clouding of the senses (blurry vision, flickering in front of the eyes, feelings of dizziness)
- Can lead to bloating/swelling (edemas)
- Leads to excessive thirst
- Leads to pimples and itching of the skin
- Can lead to nervousness and aggression

Naturally occurs in:
- Citrus fruits (lemons, limes, oranges, etc.)
- Many kinds of berries (such as red currants)
- Sea buckthorn
- Juniper
- All unripe fruits
- Pomegranate
- Sorrel
- Vinegar (apple cider vinegar is best)
- All products pickled in vinegar (sour pickles, "mixed pickles," etc.)
- All products created through lactic fermentation (yogurt, whey, kefir, etc.; be sure to use lactic bacteria that rotate to the right! Sauerkraut is also created through lactic fermentation.)

3. The Salty Taste

- Supports the body's powers of resistance
- Stimulates the appetite
- Has a heat-forming effect
- Increases the digestive heat
- Can be externally applied as salt compress (for example, on edemas and the area of the liver)
- Beneficial for the nerves (= opens the fine *Lung* channels)
- Can have an opening effect on the soul
- Cures *Lung* diseases
- Cures *Péken* diseases

Excessive intake:
- Leads to loss of hair and premature graying
- Increases formation of wrinkles
- Can lead to bad teeth
- Decreases the body strength
- Leads to excessive thirst
- Promotes swelling (edemas)
- Leads to diseases of bodily energy *Tripa* (bile)
- Leads to diseases of blood
- Can lead to hardening (also in emotional life)

Naturally occurs in:
- All naturally occurring salts (rock-salt, sea salt, soda, saltpeter, sodium nitrate, etc.) Favor sea salt since it has the same mineral distribution as human blood. If you live in an area with iodine deficiency, iodized salt is advisable.
- In foods, mainly through additional salting

4. The Bitter Taste

- Intensifies mental alertness
- Cures hoarseness
- Regulates the digestion
- Beneficial against diseases in chest area
- Beneficial against anorexia
- Can cure poisoning
- Beneficial against excessive thirst
- Has drying effect
- Cures diseases of bodily energy *Tripa* (bile)

Excessive intake:
- Increases the bodily energies *Lung* (wind) and *Péken* (phlegm)
- Consumes the bodily constituents, which can result in emaciation, dizziness, tiredness, certain deficiencies, etc

Naturally occurs in:
- Many types of lettuce (chicory, radicchio, etc.)
- Many types of vegetables and herbs (such as fenugreek, dandelion)
- Aconite (caution! very poisonous!)
- Gentian

5. The Hot Taste

- Increases digestive heat
- Stimulates the appetite
- Generally supports digestion
- Helps expand arteries and veins
- Has drying effect
- Purgative effect and intestinal cleansing (also good against worms)

- Beneficial against diseases of the throat
- Beneficial against swelling
- Cures diseases of the bodily energy *Lung* (wind)
- Cures diseases of the bodily energy *Péken* (phlegm)

Excessive intake:
- Consumes bodily strength
- Consumes semen and ovum
- Brings malaise of sensations and pain (for example, in the kidney area or the entire back; joint pain)
- Can lead to slight sense of coldness and shivering
- Can lead to loss of consciousness
- Intensifies skin irritations
- Intensifies burns
- Has drying effect on skin and mucous membranes
- Can promote aggressions and desires

Naturally occurs in:
- Primarily in spices (pepper, paprika, cloves, etc.)
- Ginger
- Garlic
- Onions
- Radishes
- Mustard

6. The Astringent Taste
- Has drying effect (for example, on bile or fat)
- Slows down the digestive heat
- Has basic slowing effect on all functions
- Beneficial against diarrhea
- Clears the complexion
- Cures diseases of the bodily energy *Tripa* (bile)

Excessive intake:
- Allows mucus to collect (tough, stringy phlegm in the bronchial tubes, for example)
- Causes bad digestion (flatulence, for example)
- Can lead to heart diseases (Roemheld's syndrome, for example)

- Lets the nutriments and bodily constituents dry out
- Generally dries up fluids
- Constricts arteries and veins (positive effect for bleeding)

Naturally occurs in:
- Rare in foods
- Unripe walnuts (very characteristic astringent taste!)
- Hamamelis virginiana (witch hazel)
- Meadow cranesbill (in medicine mixtures, for example)
- Pomegranate
- Spanish chestnuts
- Wild fruits, such as apples (also very sour)
- Acorns
- Various tree barks that are mixed into Tibetan medicines (such as sandalwood, tamarisk, acorn, Indian beech)

Here is a **chart** on the increase (= tonification) and the decrease (= pacification) of the three bodily energies through the types of tastes:

INCREASE/DECREASE OF THE BODILY ENERGIES THROUGH THE TASTES

	Increase through:	Decrease through:
Lung (wind)	Bitter	Salty
	Astringent	Sour
	Sweet/hot	Sharp/sweet
Tripa (bile)	Sour	Bitter
	scharf	Astringent
	Salty	Sweet
Péken (phlegm):	Sweet	Bitter
	Salty	Astringent
	Sour (bitter)	Hot (sour)

Many substances have various types of tastes in different proportions. In addition, the proportions should be seen as a dynamic principle and not something static. The classic example of this is rhubarb, which has a triple combination of sour, sweet, and astringent tastes. Don't become discouraged in the face of all the classifications of Tibetan medicine. Instead, this information is meant to contribute to the perspective that depicts life as an infinite learning process in the greatest variety of forms of expression.

The Secondary Reactions

The importance of the proper proportions in harmony with a possible existing imbalance of a bodily energy and/or the basic personal constitution should be emphasized once again since this is the precondition for lasting health and well-being.

But what happens when we already have an imbalance of one bodily energy and ingest too much of a balancing taste or the wrong type of taste? Two reactions may occur in this case:

1. The original imbalance remains *and* an additional imbalance of another bodily energy is added to it.
2. The original imbalance is relieved *but* an additional imbalance of another bodily energy takes its place.

Both of these imbalanced reactions can be triggered by the dietary habits and behavior patterns, as well as inappropriate medicine. In Tibetan medicine, these are called the "opposite secondary reactions *without* elimination of the existing imbalance" or "opposite secondary reactions *with* the elimination of the existing imbalance."

TO NUMBER 1 (S. ABOVE):
OPPOSING SECONDARY REACTIONS WITHOUT ELIMINATION OF THE EXISTING IMBALANCE

Existing imbalance (remains)	+ Too much of the taste	Secondary reaction imbalance (additional imbalance)
Lung/wind	Bitter	*Péken*/phlegm
Lung/wind	Hot	*Tripa*/bile
Tripa/bile	Salty	*Péken*/phlegm
Tripa/bile	Hot	*Lung*/wind
Péken/phlegm	Bitter	*Lung*/wind
Péken/phlegm	Salty	*Tripa*/bile

OPPOSING SECONDARY REACTIONS WITH
ELIMINATION OF THE EXISTING IMBALANCE

Existing imbalance (cured)	+ Too much of the taste	Secondary reaction (additional imbalance)
Lung/wind	Sweet	*Péken*/phlegm
Lung/wind	Salty	*Tripa*/bile
Tripa/bile	Sweet	*Péken*/phlegm
Tripa/bile	Bitter	*Lung*/wind
Péken/phlegm	Hot	*Lung*/wind
Péken/phlegm	Sour	*Tripa*/bile

The possibility that an additional imbalance of a bodily energy may occur should not discourage you. Instead, the information in these two charts enables us to react very precisely with the appropriate remedies to symptoms of a disrupted bodily energy that may possibly occur.

The Tastes During and
After the Digestive Phase

All ingested substances (medicines, foods, etc.) are subject to a distinct change in the stomach, small intestine, and parts of the large intestine during the digestive process. This also changes their "taste," meaning the composition of the elements within them.

The effect of a substance on one of the three bodily energies varies during this process. The types of tastes during and after the digestive phase are called the post-digestive tastes. The tastes of sweet and salty become *sweet*. The taste of sour remains *sour*, and the three remaining tastes of bitter, hot, and astringent become *bitter*.

Each of the post-digestive tastes provides relief for two bodily energies. Sweet relieves *Lung* (wind) and *Tripa* (bile), sour cures *Péken* (phlegm) and *Lung* (wind), and bitter helps reduce *Péken* (phlegm) and *Tripa* (bile).

TYPES OF TASTES AND DIGESTIVE PHASE

Taste before digestion	Taste after digestion	Cures bodily energy
Sweet and salty	Sweet	*Lung + Tripa*
Sour	Sour	*Lung + Péken*
Bitter, hot, and astringent	Bitter	*Péken + Tripa*

With the help of this chart, a finer gradation of the selected food can be created for the daily diet.

This chapter of Tibetan pharmacology also constitutes a great challenge for the Tibetan physician, who is always his or her own pharmacologist and chemist. For the effectiveness of a medicinal substance, it may be more important to have a balancing post-digestive taste than a balancing initial taste. One example of this is wood salt: Although this type of salt, which is extracted from wood, is "hot," it can be used against an excess of the bodily energy *Tripa* (bile)—because its post-digestive taste is "sweet."

We can also imagine how difficult this differentiation becomes when a great variety of substances are compounded into a medicinal combination.

The Active Powers (Potencies) of the Types of Tastes

As already mentioned in the description of the elements (see page 40f. and page 108f.), every type of taste has a characteristic quality or active power of its own. We could also call these attributes the primary quality of a healing power. These are called "potencies" in Tibetan medicine since they possess extraordinary energies. These active powers are mainly divided into the cooling qualities (= the cool nature of the moon, Tib. *gang chen*) and the warming qualities (= the warming nature of the sun, Tib. *big-dsche*). Both of these qualities are called "strengths."

There are basically eight active powers:
- Heavy
- Oily
- Cool
- Blunt
- Light
- Coarse
- Hot
- Sharp

The Tibetan language gives names to things or qualities that already contain the result. So the term "active power" can be understood both in the sense of an inherent power and the effect produced. In keeping with the first meaning, a word like "hot" can indicate that a substance has hot components; but the term can also mean that the substance has a "heating" effect.

Another example: The active quality "oily" means that oil is present as a substance. As an active power, "oily" means that the substance has a corresponding effect. The quality "blunt" describes a condition. As an active power this can also mean "pain relieving". This is not a contradiction-it rather adds certain components and therefore expands the respective view and imagination. The eight active powers therefore, can be viewed in a substantial view as well as in a view that already contains the result.

On the basis of their composition from the five elements, both the types of tastes and the active powers can also be applied for the basic constitution of each person. These can be seen on both a physical-material level and an emotional or spiritual/mental level. A person with prevailing *Tripa* energy will also have the dominant active powers of "hot," "sharp," and "oily." If we focus on the active power of "hot," we can usually assume that this person will have strongly pronounced body heat, as well as possessing a passionate emotional nature. Consequently, this person may sometimes be very quick in reacting "hotly" to a situation. Someone with a prevailing *Péken* energy may have difficulty in openly showing feelings because of the active power of "cool." These examples should give you the opportunity of observing your own personal basic constitution accordingly.

These eight active powers can be divided into four complementary pairs:
- Hot and cool
- Heavy and light
- Oily and coarse
- Blunt and sharp

The active powers can also be classified with the six types of tastes:

Heavy:	sweet	astringent	salty
Light:	bitter	sour	hot
Cool:	sweet	bitter	astringent
Hot:	salty	sour	hot
Oily:	salty	sour	sweet
Blunt:	bitter	astringent	sweet
Coarse:	sour	hot	bitter
Sharp:	salty	sour	hot

Tibetan physicians also work with a system of rating the tastes within the primary active powers and the secondary qualities. For example, the taste "sweet" is rated as extremely heavy; on the other hand, the taste "salty" is rated as not very heavy. There are various systems for this purpose that deviate somewhat from each other, but will not be described in detail within the scope of this book.

The active powers can be used in combination with the six types of tastes and the three post-digestive tastes when healing an excess of one of the bodily energies. An active power with the same qualities as the corresponding bodily energy will also increase this energy. An active power with the opposing qualities will provide relief for an excessively present bodily energy. This happens in the following manner:

Bodily energy	Increase through active powers	Relief through active powers
Lung/wind	Light, coarse, cool	Heavy, oily
Tripa/bile	Hot, hot, oily	Cool, blunt
Péken/phlegm	Heavy, oily, cool, blunt	Light, coarse, hot, sharp

The Secondary Qualities

The above-mentioned active powers represent the essence of the seventeen secondary qualities. The secondary qualities contain the eight active powers and eleven additional modes of action; these depict the inner fine-tuning of a substance or a state. Primarily when remedies are mixed, this fine-tuning can be very important.

In the daily diet, these factors tend to play a subordinate role. However, these additional qualities can clearly expand the personal experience and the perspective of every human being in the course of time. Tibetan medicine differentiates between the seventeen secondary qualities of a substance or state according to the respective degree of:

- Smoothness
- Heaviness
- Warmth
- Oiliness
- Solidity
- Coldness
- Bluntness
- Coolness
- Pliability
- Degree of fluidity (= compactness)
- Dryness
- Ability to absorb (= receptivity)
- Heat (promoting ripening)
- Lightness
- Sharpness
- Coarseness
- Flexibility

There are possibilities of differentiating within each substance or state here as well. An evaluation system (for example, from "present to an extremely strong degree" = 10 points to "present to a minimal degree" = 1 point) is used for classifying the respective secondary qualities. If we stay with the above example: The taste of "sweet" is rated within the category of "heavy" in this system with 10 points; the taste of "salty" would receive 1 point within the same category.

This fine differentiation enables a Tibetan physician to compound a medicinal composition in a way that is precisely attuned to the patient in its nuances and details. Although the differentiation system of the secondary qualities within the respective substances has been established in the medical commentaries, the Tibetan physician must still train his or her sense of taste in an extraordinary manner; depending on the different emphasis, such as the climatic circumstances, the medicinal substances will also vary in their inner fine-tuning. In addition, the physician must also include the types of tastes, the post-digestive tastes, as well as the active powers, in his or her deliberations and then balance these with the "Twenty Characteristics of Disease" (= the 17 secondary qualities plus degree of hardness, fluidity behavior, and density). If we remember that most of the Tibetan medicinal mixtures rarely contain less than two dozen different substances, then we can express our greatest appreciation of this knowledge.

General Chart of Foods
(Tastes, Active Powers, and Possibilities
of Application)

With the following charts of the various foods, you will have an additional opportunity for adapting your daily food preparation with respect to your basic constitution and/or an imbalance in one of the three bodily energies. In the last column, recommendations or commentaries regarding their use against various diseases are included. You can easily determine the effects on the three bodily energies yourself by consulting the information on the types of tastes and the active powers. Some additions have been made to the original sources—above all, there are some additional types of fruits and vegetables.

First write out a basic survey of all the foods that you like to eat. Then compare these foods with your personal basic constitution by using these charts. This will gradually give you an increasingly differentiated idea of the energetic quality of these foods. An imbalance of a bodily energy must be "treated" through the diet in the long run—so don't expect immediate success! Moreover, do not change your diet abruptly from one day to the next. Instead, "sneak" out of your current habits within the next three to four weeks. This will prevent your body—as well as your mood—from reacting too vehemently. Any long-lasting actions must also be accompanied by insight and joy.

124

Food	Taste	Active Powers	Commentary

Vegetables:

Individual vegetables are differentiated according to raw and prepared, as well as varieties that grow in dry or moist areas. Dry varieties generally have a warm and light active power; the moist varieties have a cool and heavy active power.

Food	Taste	Active Powers	Commentary
Lettuce	Bitter	Light, coarse	Difficult to digest; mainly promotes *Péken*
Tomato	Sour, sweet	Light, cool	Slightly appetite-inducing; promotes *Lung*
Sweet potato	Sweet	Heavy	Pacifying; promotes *Péken*
Potato	Sweet	Heavy, warm	Promotes *Péken*
Onion	Hot	Hot	Increases digestive heat; induces appetite: beneficial against excess of *Péken* and *Lung*; beneficial for flow of lymph (for example, when there is swelling)
Artichoke	Bitter, sweet	Light, cool	Beneficial for the liver
Asparagus	Bitter, astringent, sweet	Cool, light	Considered aphrodisiac; diuretic; good against cold lymph diseases and cold kidneys
Spinach	Bitter	Light	Difficult to digest raw; when cooked, beneficial for the liver
Chickpea	Sweet	Cool, light, absorbing	Good for expectoration and against asthma; beneficial against combined *Péken-Lung* diseases
Mushroom	Astringent	Cool, heavy	Increases *Péken*; binds poisons
Lentils	Sweet, astringent	Cool, light	Good against blood diseases; increases all three bodily energies absorbent
Peppers	Hot	Hot, coarse	Strong increasing effect on *Tripa* (and *Lung*)
Garlic	Hot	Coarse, hot, oily	Considered best medicine against excess *Lung*; cures diseases caused by microorganisms (such as worms); considered aphrodisiac; improves appetite and hair growth; good against colds, asthma, and diarrhea; weakens active

powers of medicines; closes openings of all channels; beneficial against cold *Lung* diseases of the kidneys, for example); beneficial for stomach and liver

Food	Taste	Qualities	Effects
Radish that is not fully grown, not completely ripe	Hot, somewhat bitter	Hot, coarse, light	Increases digestive heat; eliminates *Lung* diseases; beneficial against ear diseases; good for flow of lymph; external application against elephantiasis
Radish that is mature and/or stored	Hot	Heavy, warm	In raw state, increases all three bodily energies; when cooked, beneficial against excess *Lung*; both types of radish close openings of all channels and weaken active powers of medicines
Fennel	Sweetish, somewhat bitter, somewhat hot		Appetite-inducing; beneficial against excess of *Péken* and *Lung*; can reduce swelling; good for the stomach and against cold diseases
Eggplant	Sweet, bitter	Heavy	Promotes *Péken*
Cauliflower	Sweet	Heavy	Promotes *Péken*
Dandelion	Bitter, somewhat sweet	Coarse, cool	Good for detoxification in spring; beneficial against "brown phlegm" (= *Péken mugpo*)in the stomach and chronic fever; heals *Tripa* and blood diseases; beneficial against lack of appetite; appears to bind and eliminate metals
Cress	Hot	Hot, coarse	Good for strengthening health in spring; promotes *Lung* and *Tripa*
Leek	Hot	Hot	Similar to onion
Spring onion	Hot	Warm	Improves the appetite; good against combined *Péken-Lung* diseases; promotes sleep; closes the openings of all channels; unfavorable effect on medicines
Carrot	Sweet, somewhat bitter	Heavy	Promotes *Péken*; good against excess of *Lung*
Pumpkin	Sweet,	Warm	Seeds stop hot diarrhea and can be administered to promote

| | somewhat sour | | vomiting; considered "highest fruit"; beneficial for wound-healing, as well as against diseases of the lungs |

Grains:

The heaviness and coolness of grains can be changed somewhat through roasting; baking takes away more of the coolness than the heaviness. Fresh grains are generally damp and heavy; stored grains become lighter. Grains with a husk are heavier than grains without the husk.

Grain	Taste	Quality	Effects
Rice (white)	Sweet	Light, cool, smooth, oily (brown rice is somewhat heavier)	A tonic; cures all three bodily energies; good against vomiting and diarrhea; (see General Information and Preparation, on page 140)
Wheat	Sweet	Heavy, cool, oily	Beneficial against excess of Lung and/or Tripa; considered very nourishing; binds toxins in joints; good against diarrhea
Rye	Sweet	Heavy, cool	Can have balancing effect
Millet	Sweet	Somewhat heavy, cool	Good against broken bones and for wound-healing
Foxtail Millet	Sweet	Cool, light	Good against Tripa imbalance; strengthens Lung; improves appetite
Barley (with husk)	Sweet	Heavy	Outstanding tonic; increases vital fluids; provides increased peristaltic motion; (roasted barley flour boiled together with milk is beneficial against Lung)
Barley (without husk)	Sweet	Light, cool	Cures Péken and Tripa disorders; applied against formation of stones; fresh barley porridge is beneficial for the gallbladder
Buckwheat	Sweet	Cool, light	Increases all three bodily energies; good for wound-healing (external application draws blood and pus out of the wound); dissolves "blood clots"
Oat	Sweet	Heavy, hot	Strong activating effect; beneficial for the skin
Corn	Sweet	Heavy	Mitigates Lung

Milk Products:

Milk is generally heavy and cool, but becomes lighter and warmer through boiling. In Tibetan medicine, butter and fats are considered to be oils. In terms of active powers, fat is the heaviest, followed—in increasing lightness—by bone marrow, sesame oil, and butter. All oils have a sweet taste, as well as a cool, oily-fatty, and slightly laxative active power. In addition, they have smooth, blunt, and moist secondary qualities. All fats are beneficial against an excess of *Lung*. Apply externally for burns. Fats are generally beneficial for the joints.

Cow's milk	Sweet	Cool, fatty, heavy	Increases *Péken*; good for the skin; good against consumptive diseases; considered aphrodisiac; beneficial against constant urge to urinate
Cow's milk fresh from the cow (lukewarm)	Sweet	Not too heavy	"Pure ambrosia"
Butter (fresh)	Sweet	Cool, fatty, heavy	Good for complexion and skin; considered aphrodisiac
Butter (about 9 months storage period)	Sweet	Lighter than fresh butter	Beneficial against excess of *Lung*, difficulties with the memory, and mental diseases in general
Clarified butter	Sweet	Warm	Apply externally to burns; internally for excess of *Lung*
Ghee (=cleared butter)	Sweet	Warm	"Pure ambrosia"; good for all mental abilities; increases body heat; improves body strength and life expectancy
Yogurt	Sour	Coarse, cool, fatty	Improves appetite; recommended against fever on basis of an excess of *Lung*; relieves overly dry bowel movement
Cooked yogurt	Sour	Coarse, warm	Beneficial against distension and diarrhea with fever
Non-fat yogurt	Sour		Stops diarrhea; good against colds and fever; increases *Lung* (somewhat). Liquid formed on surface of yogurt has cleansing effect on the channels (such as the intestine) and helps thin the bowel movement
Kefir	Sour	Cool, light	Similar to yogurt

Goat's milk	Sweet	Cool	Beneficial against heat diseases caused by an excess of *Lung*; against thirst and fever
Sheep's milk	Sweet	Heavy	Beneficial against excess of *Lung*—caution in case of heart diseases! Very nourishing, but promotes mental dullness
Mare's milk	Sour	Balanced active power	Beneficial against diseases of the lungs; increases mental dullness
Hard cheese (like matured mountain cheese)	Sour, hot	Warm, heavy, fatty	Good against slight constipation; induces appetite; beneficial against imbalances of *Peken*
Whey	Sour	Light, astringent	Collects diseases; beneficial against flu with fever, as well as diarrhea; fresh whey improves the appetite and increases digestive heat; beneficial against diseases of the spleen and stomach, as well as tumors; cures combinations of *Lung* and *Peken*; good against slight edemas and slight poisoning; the "cheese water" cures *Peken* without simultaneously increasing *Lung* or *Tripa*
Buttermilk	Sweet, sour	Fatty, coarse	Improves the appetite; cures mild constipation; cures excess of *Peken*
Condensed milk	Sweet	Heavy	Difficult to digest or indigestible

Meat:

This survey also includes types of meat that are rarely eaten in the West since this contributes to our understanding of the energetic principles.

Most of the meats that are eaten are sweet. These are mainly differentiated according to what the animal eats, as well as where it lives.

- Animals that live in dry places = meat is light, cool, coarse = good against fever on the basis of excessive *Lung* or *Péken*
- Animals that live in damp places = meat is oily-fatty, warm, heavy = good for cold *Lung* diseases and diseases of the kidneys and stomach
- Animals that live in both places = unifies the active powers

Beef	Sweet	Light, oily	Good against fever based on an excess of *Lung*; appears to have very balanced effect
Sheep	Sweet	Fatty, warm, mild	Easily digested; improves the appetite; increases bodily constituents; good against excess of *Lung* or *Péken*
Pig	Sweet	Light, cool	Good against worms; very detrimental when there is an excess of *Lung*; beneficial against "brown phlegm" (a serious digestive disease); good against fever
Goat	Sweet	Heavy, cool	Increases all three bodily energies; helpful against burns and fever
Lamb (mutton)	Sweet	Warm, oily	Considered a tonic; improves the appetite; good against excess of *Lung* or *Péken*
Hare	Sweet	Coarse, warm	Similar to rabbit
Rabbit	Sweet	Coarse, hot	Good against diarrhea; increases digestive heat
Chicken	Sweet	Light, warm	A tonic; increases regenerative fluids; good for healing wounds
Donkey	Sweet	Warm	Good against diseases of kidneys and generally against cold illnesses; beneficial against lymphatic diseases
Horse	Sweet	Warm	Rump meat like donkey
Game (such as deer)	Sweet	Light, coarse, cool	Good against fever that accompanies an excess of *Lung* or *Péken* (same applies to mountain goats and other mountain animals)
Bone marrow	Sweet	Oily, heavy, warm	Very beneficial against an excess of *Lung* (for example, as soup)

Fish	Sweet	Oily, heavy	Improves the appetite; very advisable against diseases of stomach; promotes good vision; good against excess of *Peken*, as well as edemas; considered a tonic
Egg	Sweet	Hot, heavy	Nutritious; heats up the gallbladder; egg shells are beneficial against vomiting; the egg white is considered healing for the eyes

There are additional classifications of meat regarding:

- The sex of the animal (upper portion of male animal and lower portion of female animal are each heavier)
- Fresh meat (up to a maximum of two months) has cool active powers
- Stored meat (from about 3 months to one year) becomes warmer in its active powers and therefore more nutritious and easily digested
- Meat that has been stored for a long time (about one year) and dried in the air is very beneficial against illnesses of the bodily energy *Lung*
- Raw or frozen meat is very heavy in its active powers and extremely difficult to digest; on the other hand, the active power of meat becomes increasingly lighter and warmer when it is dried or cooked.

Spices:

Salt	Salty	Warm	Increases the digestive heat; improves the appetite; frees of old waste materials and eliminates stiffness in the body; frees blocked wind (*Lung*); too much salt lets blood and bile (*Tripa*) increase and causes loss of hair, premature graying, thirst, wrinkles, and is bad for the eyes

Substance	Taste	Quality	Effects
Sugar	Sweet	Cool	Increases *Péken*; very pacifying for *Lung*; brown raw sugar cures excessive body heat, thirst, nausea, fainting, and *Tripa* diseases
Molasses	Sweet	Warmer than sugar	Considered to be the "essence of trees"; aphrodisiac; causes emptying of intestines
Honey	Sweet	Warm	Promotes digestive heat; considered to be the "essence of the flower kingdom"; cures diseases of stomach and spleen; used as "medicinal horse" (= carrier substance) in phlegm and lymph diseases; because of its warming post-digestive taste, it can also be used in moderation by diabetics
Pepper (*black and white*)	Hot	Hot, coarse	Post-digestive taste is also hot; black pepper is considered more effective; beneficial against excess of *Péken* and cold illnesses; beneficial against difficulties with digestion; too much pepper intensifies *Lung* and *Tripa*
Pepper (*long*)	Hot, sweet	Oily, coarse	Beneficial against excess of *Lung* and cold illnesses; good against diseases of the spleen; also beneficial against an excess of *Péken*; one of the "three hot substances"; considered an aphrodisiac
Mustard seed	Hot	Relatively mild; warm, coarse	Increases *Tripa*; collects and binds toxins in the body; good against kidney and abdominal diseases, and infections; beneficial for lymph system; considered an aphrodisiac
Horseradish	Hot	Hot, light	Increases *Tripa*
Ginger	Sweet, hot	Coarse, light	Increases digestive heat, as well as body heat in general; improves the appetite; beneficial against an excess of *Lung* and *Péken*, as well as combinations of the two; serves to thin the blood
Cayenne pepper	Hot	Hot	Increases *Tripa*
Coriander (*black and white*)	Sweet, hot, astringent	Warm	Considered an "unsurpassable remedy"; beneficial against an excess of *Péken* and *Lung*; beneficial against hot phlegm in the stomach (= "brown phlegm"); improves the appetite and digestive performance; beneficial against edemas and thirst
Selinum	Hot, bitter, sweet	Oily	Cures diseases of the stomach; beneficial against cold illnesses and *Péken*

Black seed	Sweet	Oily	Good for the stomach and a cold liver; one of the eight basic remedies for the lymph system
Cumin (black and white)	Sweet, hot	Mild, oily, warm	Beneficial against cold illnesses (for example, an excess of *Péken*); good against diseases of the stomach; beneficial for the liver; one of the eight basic remedies for the lymph system; intensifies digestive heat; beneficial against hot conditions of the lungs
Caraway	Sweet	Light, mild	Beneficial against *Péken* and *Lung*; improves the appetite; good against fever of the heart (for example, "heartburn") and for the eyes; cures fever and poisoning
Cinnamon	Hot, sweet, astringent, (somewhat) salty	Hot	Increases digestive heat; beneficial against cold illnesses (above all, of the stomach and liver); good against an excess of *Lung* and diarrhea
Cardamom ("Ceylon Cardamom," larger capsules)	Bitter	Coarse, hot	Beneficial against cold illnesses (above all, those of the stomach and spleen); one of the "six good substances"; considered an extraordinary remedy" for the spleen
Cardamom ("Malabar Cardamom," smaller capsules)	Bitter, hot	Light, warm to hot	Beneficial against cold illnesses, above all, those of the kidneys; also good against an excess of *Lung*; one of the "six good substances"
Calamus root	Sharp, sweet	Coarse, hot	Increases digestive heat; beneficial against digestive disorders and slight food poisoning; good against diseases of the lymph
Licorice	Sweet	Warm, mild	Promotes opening of the channels; good for the lungs (for example, against coughing); relieves thirst
Yellowwood (a pepper)	Sharp	Coarse	Good against "hangovers"; beneficial against infections through microorganisms, as well as itching of the skin
Curcuma (turmeric)	Sweet, bitter	Hot	Good against poisoning and infections; beneficial against excessive urge to urinate

Nutmeg	Sharp, bitter	Heavy, oily, hot	Very helpful against an excess of *Lung*, as well as against diseases of the heart; one of the "six good substances"; important substance for mental difficulties; do not use when there is a kidney disease since it has a cool post-digestive taste
Clove	Sharp	Hot, coarse, dry	Called "flower of the gods"; helpful against cold illnesses and an excess of *Lung*, beneficial for the liver; among the "six good substances; an extraordinary medicine for the so-called "life channel"
Juniper	Sweet, somewhat bitter	Astringent, warm	Good against digestive diseases, as well as against cold illnesses and an excess of *Lung*, binds and collects excess bile; considered an elixir; beneficial against hemorrhoids, as well as fever of the kidneys; very good for the heart; relaxes the mind (Indian juniper is considered a holy tree)
Saffron	Sweet	Cool	Constricts openings of the channels; beneficial against excess of *Tripa* bodily energy; excellent for the liver; very good against all hot illnesses; best type of saffron is orange and very fragrant

Fruit:

Many of the kinds of fruit described here are not included in the classic Tibetan texts, which is why they have been added to the chart. Most kinds of fruit are basically sweet and sour with a cooling active power.

Grape	Sweet, somewhat sour	Cool, heavy	Similar to raisin
Raisin	Sweet	Warm, heavy	Good against diseases of the lungs
Banana	Sweet	Heavy, oily	Pacifying effect on *Lung*, can cause constipation
Watermelon	Sweet	Very heavy, very cool	Has strong cooling effect
Sea buckthorn	Sour, somewhat hot	Astringent, hot	Good against excess of *Peken*; against colic and fever; promotes mucus (= stringy phlegm) expectoration and beneficial against diseases of the lungs

133

	Taste	Quality	Effects
Coconut	Sweet	Heavy, oily	Increases *Péken* (phlegm), above all (also the mucus coat of the stomach; good against hyperpepsia
Blackberry	Sweet, sour	Astringent	Good against coughing; beneficial against excess of *Lung* with fever
Raspberry	Sweet, somewhat sour	Astringent	Similar to blackberry
Lemon	Sour	Cool, coarse	Improves the appetite; blood-cleansing effect
Peach	Sweet	Heavy, coarse	Increases *Péken*
Pomegranate	Sour astringent, sweet	Warm, oily	"Unsurpassable remedy" against diseases of digestive heat; good against cold illnesses and an excess of *Lung* and *Péken*; very beneficial against diseases of the stomach; intensifies warmth in stomach and liver; good against microorganisms (like worms)
Apricot	Sweet	Relatively balanced	Good for the skin; balancing effect on excess *Lung*; seeds are used by women against infertility; apricot oil is beneficial for hair growth; generally good for wound-healing
Rhubarb	Sour, sweet, astringent, somewhat bitter	Mild, cool, light	Good against *Péken*; beneficial against poisoning; cures heat of the small and large intestine; improves the appetite; cures edemas (lymph swelling); Tibetan name for wild rhubarb (*chu bha*) also means "lymph channels"
Cherry	Sweet, sour	Cool	Stimulates liver and bile
Date	Sweet	Heavy	Considered aphrodisiac; good against diseases of the stomach
Nectarine	Sweet	Heavy	Balancing effect on an excess of *Lung*
Mango	Sweet, somewhat sour	Heavy	Increases *Péken*; seed is used against cold illnesses of the kidneys; fruit flesh is also good for the kidneys
Grapefruit	Sweet, sour, bitter	Cool	Good against digestive complaints; stimulates the appetite; can have strongly cooling effect on organs
Apple	Sweet, sour	Heavy, cool	In raw state, primarily increases *Lung*, primarily increases *Péken* in cooked state; good for small and large intestine
Strawberry	Sweet, sour	Cool, coarse	Increases *Péken* and *Lung*; wild strawberries are good for cleansing the channels, as well as for lymph flow
Red currant	Sour	Cool	Increases *Lung*

	Taste	Quality	Effects
Pineapple	Sweet, sour	Heavy, coarse	Stimulates the appetite and digestion; beneficial for the stomach
Pear	Sweet	Heavy	Eliminates sputum; good for the lungs

Nuts, Seeds, and Oils:

"Oils" have already been described under "Milk Products." Pressed oils generally have a stimulating effect on the digestive heat and strengthen the body. In addition, they serve as an inner cleansing agent for the channels (for example, the intestine). They are considered beneficial for life expectancy in general, as well as an aphrodisiac.

	Taste	Quality	Effects
Sesame (black + white)	Sweet, (somewhat) bitter	Heavy, oily, warm	Good against *Lung* diseases; an aphrodisiac; improves hair growth (used internally and externally); one of the eight basic remedies for the lymph; improves general strength of body
Sesame oil	Sweet, bitter, hot	Heavy, oily, hot	General strengthening effect on body; overweight individuals lose weight, underweight individuals gain weight; beneficial for combinations of *Péken* and *Lung*; smoothes the skin; improves hair growth
Walnut	Sweet, astringent	Heavy, oily, hot	Stimulates *Péken* and *Tripa*, which means beneficial against *Lung*; massage with walnut oil is very good for body exhausted by *Lung*; inner part of walnut shell considered beneficial for hair growth
Peanut	Sweet	Heavy, oily, hot	Very difficult to digest
Linseed seed	Sweet, bitter	Heavy, oily, soft, smooth, warm	Good against excess *Lung*; possible usage in *Tripa* and *Péken* diseases (use in moderate amounts since the post-digestive taste is hot; can have negative effect on eyes, as well as the regenerative fluids)

Beverages and Alcoholic Drinks:

The following chart can be used to understand the basic rules:

Bodily energy	Pacified by	Stimulated by
Lung/wind	Milk	Water
Tripa/bile	Water	Alcohol
Péken/phlegm	Alcohol	Milk

Water

Tibetan medicine differentiates between the various types of water. In the classic texts, fresh rainwater is considered to be the highest quality of water.

In the Tibetan *Materia Medica*, "the eight qualities" are ascribed to rainwater. Theoretically, these eight qualities (life-sustaining, satisfying, appetite-stimulating, mind-clearing, light, pleasant-tasting, cooling, and "thin") can also be added to the water. However, the natural quality is always better.

Yet, we should keep in mind that the environmental situation of the time period in which Tibetan medicine was compiled cannot be compared with the prevailing conditions today. So water from deep wells (such as mineral water) rates fifth in Tibetan medicine, following the highly praised rainwater, melted snow, river water, and water from an open spring.

Seawater and muddy water from the forest are rated even lower. Invigorating, light water that has been exposed to sunshine, that flows and has been touched by the wind is naturally preferable to the still water or even muddy/marshy water from a dark forest.

In terms of mineral waters, there are entire libraries of differing recommendations. The experts also disagree about water filters, etc. No matter what opinion on this topic we would like to agree with, if we want to adhere to the above recommendations of Tibetan medicine, we can place our water in the sun for a certain amount of time each day, for example. This will charge it with the warming active powers of the sun's life-giving energy. Moreover, a bit of shaking may also be beneficial since water that has been standing for too long increases all three of the bodily energies in an unnatural manner. Cool water calms *Tripa* (bile), hot water stimulates the digestive heat and pacifies *Péken* (phlegm), and warm water pacifies *Lung* (wind).

Milk

Most types of milk have a sweet taste and fatty, as well as heavy and cool, active powers. Milk has a beneficial effect on the skin, increases the bodily constituents and potency, as well as the bodily energy *Péken* (phlegm). Milk generally reduces *Lung* (wind) and *Tripa* (bile). Cow's milk is considered beneficial for the lungs, as well as useful against diabetes. All of the so-called "white channels," which means certain nerve conductors starting at the brain are nourished by the bodily energy *Péken* (phlegm). In this way, milk can also have an effect on the sharpness of the mind.

The above chart lists the effects of the individual types of milk, as well as milk products. In general, restrictions should be made for all milk products in the Western industrial nations since these are very frequently saddled with added hormones and antibiotics. Some Tibetan physicians see this as a reason to warn against the excessive consumption of milk products.

Alcoholic Beverages

In terms of alcoholic beverages, we must differentiate between the alcohol produced through fermentation and distillation. Most alcoholic beverages have a sweet, sour, or bitter taste. All yeast products belong to the bodily energy *Péken* (phlegm), which means that beer made from yeast fermentation increases *Péken* (also because of its sweet taste, among other things).

A little glass of beer won't hurt a person with a predominant *Lung* constitution. On the other hand, drinks like schnapps (brandy) with its hot, thin, and slightly laxative effect can be distinctly classified as *Tripa* (bile) since they clearly increase this particular bodily energy. Consequently, a person with a predominant *Péken* constitution can also allow himself a little glass of schnapps on occasion. Freshly made spirits have a heavier active power than alcoholic drinks that have been stored and matured for years.

Wine can be classified between the two poles of beer and schnapps. Although it slightly increases the bodily energy of *Tripa* (bile), it can still be recommended occasionally after meals for a person with a *Lung* constitution. A good choice would then be a more mature red wine from the southern slopes of the mountains. Sparkling wine, champagne, and the like have a higher proportion of carbon dioxide. Since they generally have a great deal of acid in them, they mainly belong to the category of *Lung* (wind). Sweet liquors primarily increase the energies of *Péken* (phlegm), as well as *Tripa* (bile). Mixtures of various alcoholic drinks are very unhealthy. It is obvious that excessive consumption of alcoholic beverages will harm any human being. The descriptions of the consequences of excessive drinking in the Tibetan texts begin with conduct like "inconsideration and shamelessness." They say that alcohol causes "behavior like an elephant gone crazy." This ultimately leads to the "unconscious state of a corpse."

Tea

Most types of green and black tea can be classified as bitter with coarse and light active powers. They mainly increase the bodily energy of *Lung* (wind). Green tea leaves can be used as a bath additive for gouty bone fever. People with a *Lung* constitution should either avoid black tea completely or only drink it with milk.

Unfermented green tea also greatly increases the energy of *Lung*, but in a subtler manner than black tea since its secondary qualities are not quite as coarse and hard. In general, green tea has an overall strengthening effect on the body. For people with a *Péken* constitution, it is an excellent morning drink.

Herb Teas and Coffee

As a watery extract of a plant drug, all herb teas possess an effect corresponding to the respective plant. For more information see *Addresses* on page 240.

Because of its bitter taste, coffee primarily increases the bodily energy *Tripa* (bile), as well as *Lung* (wind). Coffee has the great disadvantage of spreading diseases throughout the entire body. Since Tibetan medicine mainly endeavors to gather a disease in its own location in order to eliminate it in the appropriate manner, coffee represents a clear obstacle to therapy in this respect.

Fruit Juices

Fruit juices should be classified according to their constituents. You can easily do this by consulting the "Fruit" chart above.

Most fruit juices are sweet in taste and have a heavy and cool active power. This means they correspond to a mixture of the bodily energies *Péken* (phlegm) and *Lung* (wind). Because of their high proportion of acid, citric fruits naturally primarily increase *Lung* (wind), as well as *Tripa* (bile). In any case, fruit juices from organically cultivated fruit should be favored over conventionally grown fruit.

When selecting your fruit juice, try to use the prevailing season as your guide: When apples are ripe in the later summer, then it's time for apple juice or warm applesauce. Citrus fruits are frequently too cold and coarse for the winter. Don't be swayed by the vitamin commercials on television. Instead, it's better to orient yourself to the composition of the elements in harmony with your personal constitution.

Food	Taste	Active Powers	Commentary

General Information and Preparation:

Food	Taste	Active Powers	Commentary
Rice mush, thin	Sweet	Light	Beneficial for digestion; relieves diarrhea; eliminates excess *Lung*; has warming effect on the entire body; eliminates residue after detox treatment; promotes supple channels (such as intestine)
Rice mush, medium consistency	Sweet	Somewhat heavier	Increases digestive heat; warms the body; good against general weakness; satisfies hunger and thirst; beneficial against slight constipation
Rice mush, solid consistency	Sweet	Heavy	Stimulates the appetite; beneficial against diarrhea; good against states of weakness

Adding ginger or pepper to the *rice while it cooks* can somewhat decrease the heaviness. Rice cooked in meat broth with a solid consistency is a general strengthening agent with heavy active powers. *Roasted rice* is recommended against diarrhea and broken bones.

The following statement about sweet *creamed rice* mixed with pieces of honey has been ascribed to the historical Buddha Shakyamuni. He says that this dish drives away hunger, thirst and the winds, it cleanses the bladder and helps digestion. (see *Selected Bibliography* on page 239, R. Birnbaum *The Healing Buddha*.)

Further Preparations:

Grain broth of barley	Sweet	Heavy	Reduces digestive heat; constipating effect
Grain broth of roasted grain	Sweet	Light, smooth	Easy to digest; strengthening
Grain flour, roasted	Sweet	Heavy	Considered general strengthening agent
Dumplings of roasted grain flour	Sweet	Light, smooth	A tonic; easy to digest
Meat broth	Sweet	Light, warm	Good against general weakness, emaciation, and an excess of *Lung*; general strengthening effect
Vegetable broth	Sweet	Light, warm	Tends to have a generally balancing effect, but also strengthens
Pea soup	Sweet	Cool, light, absorbing	Increases *Péken* and *Lung*; increases the appetite; cleansing effect
Noodle soup	Sweet	Light, warm	Relieves an excess of *Lung*
Garlic butter	Hot, sweet	Oily, heavy, hot	Beneficial against an excess of *Lung*; has intense cleansing effect

Improper Combination of Foods

In the nutritional teachings of Tibetan medicine, improperly combined foods are considered "poisons." This is easy to understand since the absorption of these poisons causes an intense strain on the entire organism, and the digestive heat in particular. As a result, this often leads to a great variety of diseases and imbalances of the bodily energies. The following foods are seen as incompatible with each other:

- Fish with milk
- Milk with fruit
- Fish and egg
- Cooked legumes with yogurt and/or sugar
- Alcohol with very fresh yogurt
- Frying mushrooms in mustard oil
- Chicken with yogurt
- Chicken with a mixture of honey and oils (in equal portions)
- Meat with (white) milk products
- Meat with sour alcohol
- Meat with roasted grain flour
- Milk with sour foods

In summary, the simultaneous ingestion of two different animal substances, as well as acids and starches, do not fit well together.

Western theories of nutrition also advocate separating acids and starches as much as possible. It is quite clear that it is easier for the digestive energy to deal with just one substance or one group of substances than with a meal containing many different types of tastes.

The more clearly and simply the types of tastes can be identified, the more distinct the energy information content will also be. The separation and absorption of a substance then requires less energy and can also reach the actual place of its effectiveness in an easier way.

If we imagine the various substances in the food as the different forms of information that the body must cope with, then we can understand that a simple diet safeguards it from a constant excess or confusion of information. The digestive heat can also be relieved through a simpler combination of ingredients or through the so-called "mono diet" with warm and light active powers (such as just one meal or just vegetable soup for an entire day, etc.).

Strict fasting without the ingestion of food has an intensely disarraying effect on the bodily energy *Lung* (wind). Such fasting should only be done for longer periods of time after consulting an experienced therapist.

It is also quite obvious that foods with very cold and very hot active powers combine poorly with each other. If you suffer from heartburn, shivering or feeling flushed, discomfort or something like a sense of heaviness in the stomach area, or distention of the abdomen, it is quite likely that the mixture of foods that you have eaten either generally does not fit together or does not correspond to your basic type of bodily energy. These particular symptoms can naturally also indicate the existence of a momentary imbalance of the bodily energies.

A simple, moderate, and balanced way of living is a natural law. If we orient ourselves according to these natural principles, we will feel better, even in the short run. But over time, this lifestyle is certain to be reflected as health and balance of the body and the mind.

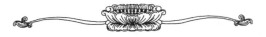

Section IV

Diagnosis in Tibetan Medicine

General Information

The diagnosis methods within Tibetan medicine have a wide-ranging spectrum of possibilities. Even without the aid of an enormous amount of technical equipment, the Tibetan physician can obtain a clear picture of the patient's condition by asking questions about the symptoms, as well as the dietary habits and behavior patterns. Careful observation of the entire body—mainly the face, the tongue, and the urine- as well as the diagnosis of the pulse are also important components of this approach.

Since Buddhism is aware of the fundamental interaction between the physical, emotional, and mental structures, Tibetan medicine also pays adequate attention to the psychological factors.

For example, the classic texts explore dream symbolism. As a result, both the conditions and the prognosis of the patient can be more clearly evaluated. Importance is also placed upon other forms of symbolism, such as interpreting the signs related to the bearer of news about an illness. The path of the physician to the patient also increases the physician's possibilities of diagnosis and prognosis.

It is truly astonishing to see how few technical aids a skilled Tibetan physician requires. Tibetan medicine represents an effective and economical medical system—just this reason alone should prompt the rich industrial nations to invest more in preserving and researching this time-honored science of healing.

Diagnosis by Questioning

Diagnosis by questioning is an important component of the Tibetan anamnesis. The Tibetan physician inquires about the life circumstances, behavior patterns, and dietary habits of the patient. After asking some additional questions, he or she can usually explain the other symptoms to the astonished patient.

The questions will not be listed individually at this point since they have been included in the corresponding chapters. Many of the respective questions have also been integrated into the short list on the personal classification with the three bodily energy types in the appendix of this book.

Basic Information about Diagnosis through the Pulse, Urine, and
Tongue, as well as the Dietary and Behavior Patterns:

If you find the characteristics listed below while examining your pulse, urine, and tongue, this always means that there is an imbalance in one of the corresponding bodily energies—usually in the form of an excess. This imbalance can then be positively influenced by means of the appropriate rules for diet and behavior.

Pulse Diagnosis

In Tibetan medicine, the pulse is considered to be a messenger that conveys information from the inside of the body to the outside world. Diagnosis by means of taking the pulse definitely represents one of the outstanding forms of diagnosis. However, it is only used in addition—but with priority—to the other diagnostic procedures.

The Tibetan form of taking the pulse is different from both the approach used by Chinese medicine and the Ayurvedic technique. The main differences are found in the position of the fingers when taking the pulse and the actual diagnosis. With this form of diagnosis, a skilled Tibetan physician is able to receive exact "data" about the entire human being. This data is in no way inferior to the so-called "hard facts" of a scientific examination.

Taking the pulse is primarily employed in evaluating the functioning/malfunctioning of the respective organs and/or their energetic equivalents. Emotional factors, mental diseases through the so-called "non-visible forces," the basic vital force ("pulse of the life basis," the *La* pulse of the ulnar artery) and much more can be comprehended through special pulse techniques. In addition, physicians also use the three death pulses, the demon pulse, the so-called illumination pulse, a family pulse, and some explicitly described pulse techniques that are generally summarized by the name of *"the seven astonishing pulses."*

However, we can assume that the pulses listed here have not been completely mastered by all Tibetan physicians. This is why they tend to be used infrequently in the practice. Yet, a skillfully performed pulse diagnosis by an outstanding Tibetan physician almost borders on clairvoyance—perhaps these abilities overlap in a life that is solely dedicated to the objective of compassion with all sentient beings and achieving a transparent state of enlightenment.

I am personally aware of the case of a patient who, according to the diagnosis of orthodox medicine, had only six months to live. Fortunately, he consulted a prominent Tibetan physician-healer. During the pulse diagnosis, the physician asked the patient about a visit to Tibet and a "souvenir" in the form of a stone that he had taken with him. But the patient had told the physician nothing at all about this beforehand! Among other things, the diagnosis and simultaneous treatment consisted of bringing the stone back to its original spot. Apparently, "non-visible forces" were involved in the man's illness to a considerable degree. Through the ritual of returning the "souvenir," as well as the appropriate recitations and so forth, it was possible to once again pacify these forces. As far as I know, this man is still alive and enjoys good health.

By using the so-called "*family pulse*" (also called "representative pulse"), a skillful physician can also make a prognosis for the illness of a patient who is not in the room through the pulse of a relative. However, the relative whose pulse is measured should be healthy. In addition, there are pulse techniques that solely serve the purpose of divination.

As already mentioned, these examples in no way represent the generally common practices within a medical consultation. They are merely meant to show the dimensions of possibilities that can be many times superior to the purely apparatus-based diagnostics of a laboratory. Moreover, the pulse diagnosis has the advantage that it is always "on hand," so to speak. Precise knowledge about the theoretical perceptions, as well as a great wealth of experience, must naturally form the basis for this type of diagnosis.

However, this introduction to Tibetan medicine is primarily meant to explore the characteristics of the three basic constitution pulses, as well as the possibilities of recognizing the three bodily energies of *Lung* (wind), *Tripa* (bile), and *Péken* (phlegm). By means of refining the sensory perception, as well as with much practice and endurance, it is possible—to a certain degree—for every human being to feel these pulses and classify himself/herself with the respective constitution type and/or determine an excess of a certain bodily energy. However, the refined form of the pulse diagnosis can ultimately only be learned under the direction of an experienced Tibetan physician.

Technique of Taking the Pulse

The *optimal time of the day for examining* the pulse is considered to be when the cold energies of the night and the warm energies of the day balance each other—the time just before the sunrise. However, the patient should not go to bed too early or too late the night before, as well as not engaging in sexual activities, drinking alcohol, or consuming foods that are difficult to digest. He should also have an empty stomach, if possible. Incidentally, these rules also apply to the physician. In addition, the patient should also not worry too much about the examination.

The traditional texts describe an optimal state in this regard. Of course, the pulse diagnosis is also possible during any other time of the day. But the physician must then also take into consideration the prevailing energy of the respective time. In the more subtle form of diagnosis by means of taking the pulse, the energies of the prevalent season should also be observed (see chart below).

There are various *areas of the body* where the pulse can be taken. However, this primarily occurs on the radial artery *(Arteria radialis)* of the lower arm. This is the bloodstream of the thumb side. This spot is considered to be at an optimal distance from the place of observation and the organs to be observed. In order to illustrate this concept, it is compared with a rushing stream. When two people are too close to this stream, they cannot carry on a conversation with each other. This would correspond approximately with taking the pulse on the neck or heart. In this case, the organs would be "too loud." But if a bloodstream is selected that is too far away from the organs (such as the hollow of the knee, behind the ankle, etc.), this would be comparable to a person who attempts to talk with you from the other side of the stream. The only exception to this rule is for children under the age of two. Their pulse is taken on the vein of the ear.

The physician and the patient sit facing each other on the same level during the pulse diagnosis. For a woman, the Tibetan physician first takes the pulse on her right arm with his left hand and then the pulse on her left arm with his right hand. For a male patient, the physician proceeds in the opposite manner. In the Tantric texts, the left side is classified with the feminine aspect, as well as the aspect of wisdom, while the right side is associated with the aspect of the methods and "the proper means." By establishing contact in a polar manner, the physician appears to create a favorable field for the patient's recovery.

The index, middle, and ring fingers are used for taking the pulse. The areas where these fingers are placed are found by leaving the space of a finger (preferably the thumb) between the little bone facing the thumb (Processus styloidens radii = styloid process of the radius) and the first finger (the index finger) placed on the arm.

The space between the index finger and the middle finger or the middle finger and the ring finger should be that of "one grain of rice," meaning that the fingers still lightly touch each other. The fingers are placed flatly and the pressure used varies with respect to the individual finger. The index finger remains on the surface, meaning the skin. The middle finger is pressed a bit deeper into the musculature, and the ring finger is pressed in very deeply, almost to the bone. This results in the *three different levels* of taking the pulse.

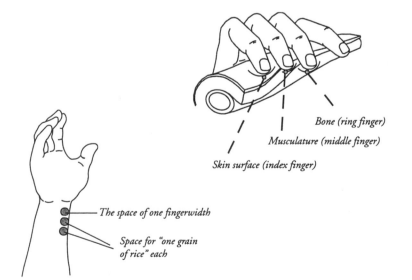

Bone (ring finger)

Musculature (middle finger)

Skin surface (index finger)

The space of one fingerwidth

Space for "one grain of rice" each

Constitutional Pulse

The primary consideration should be to find the generally prevailing pulse of an individual. This pulse, felt on the healthy person, is called the *constitutional pulse*. It is very important for a physician to know this pulse since this basic pulse could otherwise be confused with cold diseases (in the case of a "Bodhisattva pulse") or with heat diseases (in the case of a masculine or feminine pulse). If you would like to determine your own pulse, then please do this during a phase in which you feel healthy. However, you can basically discover imbalances of *Lung* (wind), *Tripa* (bile), or *Péken* (phlegm) without this pulse determination. Don't let yourself be confused at the beginning by the many different qualities of the pulse. The simplest method is to first learn the basic characteristics of *Lung* (wind), *Tripa* (bile), and *Péken* (phlegm) by heart. Then you can also learn the constitutional pulse.

- *Masculine constitutional pulse*: Is associated with *Lung* (wind). Described as coarse or rough, as well as massive or full. Women with a masculine constitutional pulse seem to have a tendency of giving birth to boys.

- *Feminine constitutional pulse:* Is associated with *Tripa* (bile). It is described as thin or fine and fast. Men with a feminine constitutional pulse appear to primarily father girls.

- *Neutral constitutional pulse* (also called the "Bodhisattva pulse", but this description should not be interpreted in the spiritual sense): Is associated with *Péken* (phlegm) and described as smooth and gentle, as well as continuous. People with this pulse appear to be ill less frequently and have a long life span.

In the *Final Tantra*, the result of marriage between two people with masculine constitutional pulses is described as primarily the conceiving of boys. The marriage of two people with feminine constitutional pulses appears to tend toward producing girls.

If the man has a pulse neutral constitutional pulse and the woman has a masculine constitutional pulse, a boy will be conceived. If the woman has a neutral pulse and the man has a feminine constitutional pulse, the result of this is conceiving a girl.

This form of diagnosis should be handled in a very subtle manner and is consequently also difficult to make. Because of this, it should only be done by an experienced Tibetan physician. Above all, the basic division into a masculine, a feminine, and a neutral constitutional pulse is important. With some practice and patience, you can learn to determine this pulse on your own.

The Pulses of the Bodily Energies
Lung (Wind), Tripa (Bile) and
Péken (Phlegm)

With a some ability, these fundamental characteristics of the corresponding constitutional pulse or an excess of the respective energy can be differentiated from each other within a relatively short period of time. Then they can also be employed together with the other diagnostic possibilities.

Lung (Wind)

A person with prevailing *Lung* energy and/or an excess of *Lung* will have the following basic pulse characteristics:

- floating or drifting
- empty
- halting
- oscillating

The wind pulse is more likely to be found on the surface and proves to have less substance, meaning that it doesn't appear to be very powerful. The quality of *floating* or *drifting* can be compared with a piece of wood on the ocean waves. The wood is thrown around from one place to the next. So the *Lung* pulse changes the place where it is felt. Another example would be imagining a water skipper that suddenly changes the place where it is hovering. A certain unpredictability or moodiness comes to light here. However, we should keep in mind that this change of place always occurs on the same level.

The pulse quality of *empty* means both that this pulse does not appear to be particularly powerful and also that there is an "empty" artery when we attempt to find the pulse by pressing the finger down more firmly. In this case, the artery is said to be "empty of the pulse." If we release the pressure of the finger somewhat, the pulse will come back again within a short time. This is like a floating ball that is held beneath the surface of the water. It has practically no basis and disappears, so it is "empty." But if we let it go, it will immediately return to the surface.

The quality of *halting* refers to both the slightly inhibited appearing energy of the pulse and the variation of its regularity, meaning that it is arrhythmic. A beat may also occasionally be missing or an additional pulsation may occur between the normal beats (*extrasystole*). The frequency in which this missing or addition beat occurs can vary greatly—in one person it may occur every three beats, in the other every thirty beats.

A further meaning of "halting" is related to the fact that the pulse beat is not completely missing, but that it hits a different point of the fingertip—it changes its location. The meaning is associated with the quality of the pulse beat: each pulse beat hits another place on the finger so that two subsequent pulse beats never hit exactly the same place on the finger.

The pulse quality *oscillating* is understood to be the hitting of the pulse beat first on one side and then on the other side of the same finger. We could also say that it "swings back and forth," but the pendulum is reversed, like a metronom—it points upward. This pulse quality is frequently also mentioned as a differentiated quality of "halting."

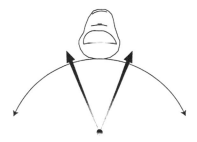

Tripa (Bile)

The pulse qualities one of person dominated by the bodily energy *Tripa* and/or an excess of the energy *Tripa* are:

- prominent
- taut or tense
- wiry
- fine (thin)
- rapid

The first pulse quality that should basically be looked for is a characteristic of the *Tripa* pulse—namely, **rapid**. The quality is relatively easy to feel. All that is required is a measurement against which "quick" can be gauged. This measurement is the length of the physician's(!) inhalation and exhalation frequency. Count the pulse beat from the beginning of the inhalation to the end of the exhalation.

During such a frequency phase, exactly five pulse beats should naturally be counted. This would then be neither a hot nor a cold disease; however, a different pulse quality indicating an excess may be discovered.

If more than five pulse beats occur, this is a heat disease, meaning an excess of the bodily energy *Tripa* or blood. Hot diseases can also arise through a combination of *Tripa* or blood with *Lung*. The higher the number rises, the greater the excess. Six or a maximum of seven beats is probably still an acceptable pulse frequency. Furthermore, we can discover how acute the disease is by counting the number of pulse beats. The same applies to a lower number of beats. This means that the fewer number of beats you count, the colder the disease is. Cold diseases can generally be associated with the *Lung* or the *Péken* energy or with a combination of *Lung/Péken*. The chronicity of an illness can also be determined on this basis.

The simplest classification of illness is into the categories of "hot" and "cold." This classification is done according to the method described above. The only conditions that can either prove to have a hot or a cold character are diseases of the lymph fluid and diseases caused by microorganisms (viruses, bacteria, worms, etc.) The number of occurring pulse beats is always a good starting point and also provides a good opportunity to "approach" the pulse during the first one to two minutes.

"We don't have to look for a *Tripa* pulse—it shows up completely on its own." This quote from Dr. Barry Clark says almost everything about the *Tripa* pulse. It comes out of the artery in an extraordinarily powerful way, so it is *prominent*. This quality can intensify into a type of boxing against the artery wall.

In addition, imagine the *tautly* tensed string of a well-tuned instrument. The more you attempt to stretch this string, meaning pressing the pulse into the depths, the stronger the resistance of the string—the resistance pushing against you from the pulse—will become. Expressed in mathematical terms, we could probably say that the resistance grows in proportion to the pressure of the finger. Yet, the string has a certain flexibility and, to a certain extent, gives way to your pressure. This pulse "flees" around the feeling finger because the tension is very high.

Moreover, the secondary pulse qualities ascribed to the bodily energy *Tripa* (bile) are *wiry*, *wound up* (within itself), and *angular*.

Péken (Phlegm)

The pulse of an individual with a *Péken* constitution and/or an excess of *Péken* can be recognized by the following characteristics:

- sunken and indistinct
- weak
- cumbersome (ponderous)

The quality of "*sunken*" refers to the level of the pulse, meaning that the pulse is sunken in the depths. This pulse can only be perceived indistinctly or even not at all on the surface of the artery. As a result, it represents almost the opposite of "protruding." Pressure must frequently be used to find the pulse. Even in the depths of the artery, this pulse can often only be perceived in a very unclear manner.

The next pulse quality reflecting an excess of *Péken* (phlegm) is *weak*. This word should be understood literally here. However, this quality could also be interpreted to mean vulnerable.

Imagine a massive and somewhat clumsy elephant that lumbers as it walks, and then you will know what *cumbersome* or *ponderous* means in terms of the pulse. This pulse has something thick or tough about it—like a soup that has boiled for too long. In addition, we could perhaps also speak of "trampling" or "wallowing" here.

Summary:		
Lung (Wind)	*Tripa* (Bile)	*Péken* (Phlegm)
Floating	Protruding	Sunken
(Drifting)	Tautly tensed	Weak
Empty	Wiry	Cumbersome
Halting	Fine	
Oscillating	Quick	

The Pulse of the Organs

In Tibetan medicine, the various organs and/or their energetic equivalent are specifically diagnosed within the examination by means of taking the pulse. For this purpose, each of the flatly placed fingers are divided into a left and a right half so that a total of twelve areas of touch are available.

The "upper" sections facing the thumb are used for the diagnosis of the vital or full organs (heart, liver, lungs, spleen, and the right and left kidney). The "lower" sections are used for the diagnosis of the hollow organs (large intestine, gallbladder, small intestine, urinary bladder, and life vessel).

There have been many discussions about the so-called "life vessel." Some authorities assume this means the seminal vesicle or the reproductive fluids (semen and ovum). On the other hand, others believe that it has no physical equivalent. According to this perspective, it would most closely correspond to a portion of the hormonal system.

The life vessel may correspond to the triple warmer of Chinese medicine since it also has its equivalent in the hormonal system. To add to the confusion, there are two different traditions of teachings within Tibetan medicine. While the one tradition assumes that the reproductive fluids represent the most refined portion within the body, the other tradition considers these fluids the "waste products" of a connected, even finer energy. Whether this subtle energy is a hormone, for example, or a non-material energy certainly cannot be definitively explained here.

The full organs should basically have more attention paid to them since they are directly related to the seasonal qualities. But, as a result, they may also be easily confused with these qualities (see page 161ff.)

Furthermore, keep in mind that the organs of the woman and of the man exchange places on the left and right of the physician's index finger (see illustration below). This is related to the different dominance of the channels in the corresponding sex. Even in the West, we generally speak of one side as more "feminine" and the other as more "masculine." However, this is explained on the basis of the different functions of both brain hemispheres.

The following organs are palpated on the inside of the left arm:
- With the physician's index finger: lungs and large intestine in a woman, heart and small intestine in a man
- With the physician's middle finger: spleen and stomach
- With the physician's ring finger: left kidney and life vessel

Left radial artery
"Upper" palpation, which means facing the physician's thumb:
    1 Lungs (in a woman)
    1 Heart (in a man)
    2 Spleen
    3 Left kidney

"Lower" palpation, which means facing toward the physician's little finger:
    4 Large intestine (in a woman)
    4 Small intestine (in a man)
    5 Stomach
    6 Reproductive fluids (life vessel)

The following organs are palpated on the inside of the right arm:

- With the physician's index finger: heart and small intestine in a woman, lungs and large intestine in a man
- With the physician's middle finger: liver and gallbladder
- With the physician's ring finger: right kidney and urinary bladder

Right radial artery

"Upper" palpation, which means facing the physician's thumb:

1 Heart (in a woman)
1 Lungs (in a man)
2 Liver
3 Right kidney

"Lower" palpation, which means facing toward the physician's little finger:

4 Small intestine (in a woman)
4 Large intestine (in a man)
5 Gallbladder
6 Urinary bladder

The full organs each have additional pulse qualities that correspond to them. These are explicitly described in the *Final Tantra*. This will not be discussed here in detail since they are the object of a very subtle form of pulse diagnosis, which can easily take one to two years to learn.

The basic problem with these organ pulses is primarily that there is no exact measurement against which these qualities can be gauged. Consequently, it is only possible for them to be communicated by a Tibetan physician.

It usually takes at least several months for a person to master the above pulse qualities and distinctions between the organs. So too much information at this point would tend to lead to confusion instead of additional knowledge of the pulse diagnosis.

Classification of the Individual Organs with the Elements

The individual organs are associated with the following corresponding elements:

Element	Organ
• Wood (= air)	Liver and gallbladder
• Fire	Heart and small intestine
• Earth	Spleen and stomach
• Metal (= iron)	Lungs and large intestine
• Water	Kidneys and urinary bladder

This results in the association of the elements with the corresponding fingers, upon which the organs for taking the pulse are located.

Finger (Left Hand)	Element		Finger (Right Hand)	Element
1 Index finger	Iron		4 Index finger	Fire
2 Middle finger	Wood		5 Middle finger	Earth
3 Ring finger	Water		6 Ring finger	Water

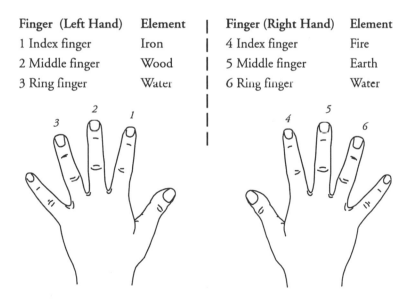

Since a different element prevails during each season, the respective corresponding organs are also influenced accordingly (also see *Seasonal Changes*, on page 72f., for information on seasons as direct causes). In the pulse diagnosis, this is mainly expressed through a more distinct movement of the correlating organ pulses. If the organ pulse is expressed in keeping with the prevailing season, this is evaluated as a positive sign. However, the seasonal qualities can also be palpated under all of the fingers.

There are various divisions for the course of the Tibetan year. In the chart below, the beginning of the Western spring lies exactly in the middle of the Tibetan spring and the beginning of the Western autumn lies exactly in the middle of the Tibetan autumn. The other seasons can be deduced directly from this fact. The chart below basically harmonizes with the seasons that prevail in the West. Each season lasts 72 days. A phase of 18 days, during which the spleen pulse and the earth element rule, is inserted between each normal season.

WESTERN SEASONS AND ELEMENTS

Spring: The ruling element is wood
The liver pulse is more distinct (fine and taut)

Summer: The ruling element is fire
The heart pulse is more distinct (full and slower)

Autumn: The ruling element is metal (iron)
The pulse of the lungs is more distinct (short and coarse)

Winter: The ruling element is water
The kidney pulse is more distinct (slow and soft)

Phases in between: The ruling element is earth
The pulse of the spleen is more distinct (short and soft)

This division of the seasons can easily be translated into our seasons. However, two different systems for dividing the year should also be mentioned here for the sake of completeness:

1. Division of the seasons in such a way that the above in-between phases are integrated into the one season of "late summer."

2. Division into six climatic periods lasting two months each:

Spring (March/April = 1st and 2nd month)
Late Spring, Early Summer (May/June = 3rd and 4th month)
Summer corresponds with the Monsoon (July/August = 5th and 6th month)
Autumn (September/October = 7th and 8th month)
Early Winter (November/December = 9th and 10th month)
Late Winter (January/February = 11th and 12th month)

(Note: These months correspond with the seasons in the Northern Hemisphere.)

The Reciprocal Influences of the Elements

The following rules apply to the reciprocal influencing of the elements:

1. The mother-child cycle

2. The friend-enemy cycle

The Mother-Child Cycle
The mother cycle refers to the generating qualities of an element in relation to the element that is "lower" in the vertical series.

Wood (air) is the mother of fire—fire is the mother of earth—earth is the mother of iron (metal)—iron (metal) is the mother of water—water is the mother of wood (air).

A child cycle can also be read in this chart by reading from bottom to top: water is the child of iron (metal)—iron (metal) is the child of earth—earth is the child of fire—fire is the child of wood (air)—wood (air) is the child of water.

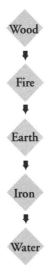

The Friend-Enemy Cycle

This cycle is related to the respective inhibiting or supporting elements in relation to each other. The elements are written in a horizontal row for this purpose:

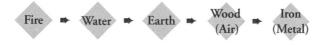

The enemy cycle (= inhibition) is read from left to right. This means that the enemy of fire is water—the enemy of water is earth—the enemy of earth is wood (air)—enemy of wood (air) is iron (metal)—the enemy of iron (metal) is fire.

The Friend Cycle

The friend cycle (= support) is read from right to left. This means that the friend of iron (metal) is wood (air)—the friend of wood (air) is earth—the friend of earth is water—the friend of water is fire—the friend of fire is iron (metal).

When summarizing all of the above cycles, they are written with both rows together:

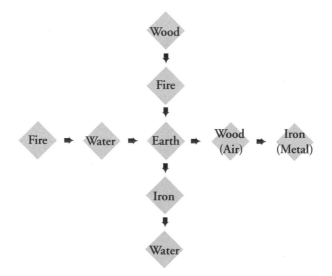

By using the mother-child cycle, as well as the friend-enemy cycle, we can recognize through which organs we can indirectly influence the organ to be treated. For example, this allows the direct strain on an organ in a heated condition to be reduced, etc. This naturally results in a great variety of therapeutic consequences and possibilities.

The energy theory depicted above appears to be related to the teaching of the five elements in Traditional Chinese Medicine. It may also be that the aspects of pulse diagnosis, as well as the element theory, come from Chinese medicine and have been integrated into the Tibetan system in the appropriately modified form.

A very lovely Tibetan illustration on this topic is found in the *Fundamentals of Tibetan Medicine* by Tsewasng J. Tsarong:

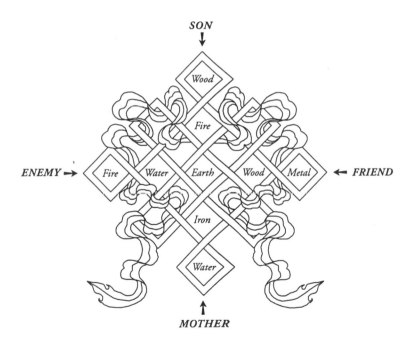

The Tibetan pulse diagnosis represents a form of diagnosis that is difficult to master. Yet, with intuition and endurance, we can learn it ourselves to a substantial degree. In addition to the other diagnostic procedures, it can become a very valuable aid.

The effort and exertion related to learning this form of diagnosis is certainly worth it. Moreover, the pulse diagnosis offers a wonderful opportunity for intensifying and refining our own personal perceptive abilities.

Urine Diagnosis

The urine of a human being represents an excellent diagnostic medium. It clearly reflects all of the metabolic processes in the body.

Even in the West, there used to be a so-called "traditional urinoscopy," which unfortunately no longer exists in its original form. The direct lineages reflecting how this form of diagnosis was handed down end at the beginning of the historic period called the "Enlightenment." A modified form of this classic diagnosis procedure is still done today—mostly by naturopaths—using various reagents, overlays, etc. However, there is a substantial difference between this Western approach and the methods described here.

Tibetan urinoscopy can certainly be used at least as an additional criteria for this purpose. But it also offers anyone who is interested the opportunity of attaining a very good overview of the digestive and metabolic processes, meaning the condition of the bodily energies.

The basic requirement for this form of diagnosis is a medium amount (approx. 150-250 ml) of urine that has been voided in the morning of the same day. Some Tibetan physicians prefer the mid-stream urine, but it doesn't appear to be absolutely necessary. If we divide the entire amount of morning urine into three "portions," then the second urinary stream is the mid-stream urine.

In the traditional texts, any urine voided after midnight is considered to be acceptable for the examination. However, this statement is based on the habits of people in earlier times who went to bed at the latest shortly after the sun set. This means that a number of hours, during which the urine could accumulate, had passed by midnight. In our present age with artificial lighting, etc., the time at which people go to bed is probably much later so that only the morning urine fulfills the corresponding criteria for the examination. If you get up during the night to snack on something from the refrigerator or to urinate, the morning urine cannot be used for diagnostic purposes.

It is naturally best to immediately examine the fresh urine. However, this urine can still offer very good examination results up to the evening of the same day. It can basically even be used for up to a total of 24 hours after voiding. Since there are frequently great distances to be bridged in Tibet and the Himalayas when a person needs to see the doctor, there are special examination techniques for cold urine, but these will not be described here.

The technical equipment required for this diagnosis consists of a white vessel that is not too large (such as a pot made of porcelain) in which the visual aspects of the urine are clearly visible, as well as a long wooden stick (about 8 inches long) to stir the urine.

In order to guarantee an optimal diagnosis, observe the following *preparatory measures*:

- Food supplements and additionally ingested vitamins interfere with the color of the urine. It would be best to stop taking them one week before the diagnosis. Otherwise, the color could indicate conditions like a latent fever or pregnancy.
- Foods that have a strong coloring effect, like red beets, can be confused with blood in the urine. Eliminate them from your diet at least one day before.
- Sexual activities can lead to confusion about conditions like kidney insufficiency, so at least abstain from them on the evening before.
- Do not drink alcohol the evening before the urine diagnosis. This could be mistaken for an imbalance of the bodily energy *Tripa* (bile).
- On the day before, avoid any type of excess as much as possible. This means not exerting yourself too much, not eating too late in the evening, and not eating fatty foods. Go to bed at a moderate time.

- If you must go to the toilet at night, then you can't use the morning urine! Only use the urine that you have collected during the entire night and in the morning for the diagnosis.
- If you do snack on something from the refrigerator during the night, the morning urine will not provide adequate information.

Evaluation Criteria in Urine Diagnosis

All the factors of color, smell, consistency, formation of bubbles, and contents are used to evaluate the morning urine. The behavior of the urine over a longer period of time—such as the observation of how various surface layers of fatty substances are formed, the development of certain patterns, or the so-called albumen (a substance that mostly provides information about the bile flow and the functioning of the liver) for diagnostic and divinatory purposes (uromancy)—is beyond the scope of this book. I will only mention that the divination is done by mentally projecting the pattern of a turtle shell onto the cooled urine, for example. Needless to say, this requires a great deal of experience.

The general criteria for recognizing the imbalances of one of the bodily energies is described in the following section:

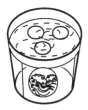

Urine when there is a Lung (wind) imbalance

The color of this urine is described as transparent as mountain water and pale. When there is a chronic *Lung* imbalance, a slightly pale blue color may be observed. The urine has practically no smell at all and possesses a fine, light and thin, almost watery consistency. When this urine is stirred with a wooden stick, bubbles up to the size of a silver dollar form on the surface. These bubbles are traditionally described as being "as large as a yak's eye." These bubbles may also have a bluish shimmer to them. No steam develops during urination.

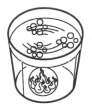

Urine when there is a Tripa (bile) imbalance

The color of this urine ranges from dark yellow to reddish orange. In a mixture with an imbalance of the blood, it may even assume an almost reddish color. In the case of hepatitis (inflammation of the liver), the color even resembles a strong black tea or a cola drink.

When an excess of *Tripa* exists, the smell is putrid in the worst case. But, in any case, it is always clearly perceptible. The consistency is more viscous and thick than in an excess of *Lung*. There are little bubbles on the surface, which burst after a short time. These bubbles may also develop when the urine is stirred. Because of the heat present, they cannot form any type of stability. This urine also shows a strong development of steam, which also remains for some time. In a chronic *Tripa* imbalance, hanging, half-transparent formation that resembles cotton may float in the urine. (These are called *guja* in Tibetan, probably a formation from the albumen.) The position in the urine corresponds with that of the *Tripa* imbalance in the body. For example, if it hangs in the center of the urine specimen, this means an imbalance in the middle body area.

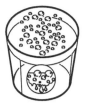

Urine when there is a Péken (phlegm) imbalance

This urine displays a pale and watery to gray color. In the extreme case, this can intensify to a milky coloration. The formation of bubbles on the surface is reminiscent of foam created when beer is poured too vehemently. At latest, these bubbles occur when the urine is stirred. They are very static and also remain for a long period of time. The consistency and location of the foam only changes after some time. This may even take several minutes. There will hardly be any smell from this urine specimen, and practically no steam will develop during voiding. In its composition and smell, the urine in a *Péken* imbalance is similar to the urine described under "*Lung*/Wind," but it isn't as thin and watery and as pale and transparent.

The following *charts* list the individual criteria as an aid in orientation:

Color
- Transparent to pale blue: indicates a *Lung* imbalance
- Yellow to orange: indicates a *Tripa* imbalance
- Pale to whitish: indicates a *Péken* imbalance
- Rainbow color: indicates poisoning
- Yellow to red: imbalance of *Tripa* and/or blood (heat disease)
- Pale and blue: imbalance of *Lung* and/or *Péken* (cold disease)
- Pink to red: imbalance of blood (and/or menstruation)
- Greenish: may indicate a possible pregnancy
- Copper-colored (shiny): indicates a latent fever
- Color like black tea or a cola drink indicates liver inflammation

Formation of Bubbles
- Bubbles the size of silver dollars with a bluish shimmer indicate a *Lung* imbalance

- Small bubbles that burst with a pop after a while indicate a *Tripa* imbalance
- Formation of foam like poured beer indicate an excess of *Péken*; the bubbles are static
- A rainbow-like shimmer in the foam indicates poisoning
- A reddish color of the foam indicates a disease of the blood

Consistency

- Clear and light, watery, indicates *Lung*
- Slight viscosity or thickness indicates *Tripa* and/or a hot disease
- Milky and light indicates *Péken*

Development of Steam

- No or little development of steam for *Lung* and *Péken*; generally applies to all cold diseases
- Strong development in an imbalance of *Tripa;* generally in hot diseases

Smell

- No smell in *Lung*
- Strong to putrid smell in *Tripa*
- No smell to slight smell in *Péken*
- Smell like cabbage, meat, and the like (food in general) indicates too little digestive heat (or did you eat something very late the evening before?)

Contents

- Pink or red "dots" indicate an imbalance of the blood or menstruation
- Floating, half-transparent threads that look like vertically hanging cotton indicate a chronic *Tripa* imbalance
- "Particles" (similar to fine sand or very fine pebbles) that are floating or resting on the bottom indicate the coldness and weakness of the kidneys

You can test yourself for an imbalance of your bodily energies with this examination method, which is relatively easy to carry out. Even if you find just one of these characteristics, this is enough to verify the corresponding imbalance. However, mixed forms of the above characteristics are frequently found. Then you can attempt to discover the main tendency and accordingly adapt your behavior patterns and dietary habits. With some practice, by using your morning urine you can very precisely check to see how well you tolerated the foods that you "enjoyed" the day before. Incidentally, healthy urine smells like "old leather."

Although Tibetan medicine is familiar with auto-urotherapy, it does not discuss it in a detailed form. It appears to have been primarily used as a form of immunostimulation by physicians who had to go to an area in which an infectious disease was raging without the appropriate amount of time to prepare for it.

Tongue Diagnosis

Tongue diagnosis or the visual observation of the tongue tends to play a subordinate role in Tibetan medicine. However, it can be employed as a quick form of additional diagnosis to verify a set of symptoms.

The tongue will display the following characteristics when there is an imbalance:

Tongue when there is an imbalance of Lung (wind):
- Red
- Dry
- Little bumps at the edges
- Coarse

Tongue when there is an imbalance of Tripa (bile):
- (Pale)-yellowish coating (more or less thick)
- Slightly bitter taste
- Somewhat dirty appearance

Tongue when there is an imbalance of Péken (phlegm):
- (Pale) whitish-gray coating (more or less thick)
- Moist-sticky

- Creates a slightly "filled up," swollen impression
- Smooth surface
- Dull surface

Additional Diagnostic Possibilities

The following additional diagnostic possibilities are also described in the *Tantras*.

Division into hot and cold diseases by means of the lower eyelid:
If we slightly pull down the lower eyelid, then the skin that becomes visible will appear to be either reddish to red, which indicates a warm to hot disease, meaning an imbalance of *Tripa* (bile) and/or blood. Or it indicates a combination of *Tripa* with *Lung*. On the other hand, if the skin tends to appear pale and whitish, which indicates a cold disease, this indicates an imbalance of *Péken* (phlegm) or a combination of *Péken* and *Lung*.

Diagnosis by means of the ear veins:
If, using slight backlighting, we look from behind at the place between the mastoid (a little elevated spot at the back of the head near the ear that is very easy to feel) and the earlobe, a slight yellowish coloring may be observed. This indicates the presence of a *Tripa* imbalance.

Section V

Therapeutic Measures

Order of Priority for the Therapeutic Measures

The order of the therapeutic measures in Tibetan medicine has been clearly established:

1. Changing the dietary and behavior patterns according to the disease—in case this is inadequate:

2. Administration of medicinal substances (mainly pills, powders, or teas)—in case this is inadequate:

3. External forms of therapy—if necessary:

4. Additional possibilities through exerting a spiritual influence (done only by the lamas, not by the physician)

As you can see, the external therapeutic procedures presented here are only employed by a Tibetan physician as the last possibility since they are considered to have a relatively drastic influence on the body.

Some of these external procedures are also used in naturopathic practices, but frequently in a changed, usually much more gentle form. Except for certain exercises to promote relaxation such as *Kum Nye* (see *Selected Bibliography* on page 240) and some lighter forms of massage, they do not belong in the hands of lay people since their false application would cause more harm than good.

It is inadvisable to use the supposedly "simpler" methods like moxabustion, deeper massage, or the so-called "chakra healing" (with or without gemstones) without first undergoing qualified instruction. Although the body is definitely able to regenerate itself as long as it has enough leeway to compensate and can balance itself, don't overdo it since health is a great treasure! In the manifestation of an illness, the leeway for the body's compensation has frequently already been used up. This means it is time for a change in the dietary and behavior patterns—and for a qualified treatment.

In addition to the immense size of the third medicine tantra, the "Oral Instruction Tantra," the main reason given for not translating it into a Western language has been that the practical treatment methods can only be passed on in a proper and responsible manner under the supervision of an experienced physician. Medicine is an empirical science—if you aren't fortunate enough to have a Tibetan physician living around the corner from you, then trust in the experience of someone offering naturopathic treatment in terms of the therapies described in the following. These therapies are definitely also employed within Western naturopathy in a responsible form that is helpful to the patient.

Therapy Through Behavior and Dietary Patterns

How the diet should be changed when there is an excess of *Lung* (wind), *Tripa* (bile), or *Péken* (phlegm) has already been discussed in detail in *Dietary Habits* on page 98f.

The behavior patterns of the individual bodily energies in terms of the seasonal changes can also be found in the respective chapter (see page 93f.). In a very general way, the recommendations are valid for a basic constitution and against an excess of a bodily energy. Such an excess may also just be a temporary occurrence and only exist for a short time. So once you have made a decision, you do not have to stick with it. Remain flexible. Only through the precise observation of all the factors can optimal dietary and behavior patterns be achieved. The following summaries can be helpful in this process:

When There Is an Excess of *Lung* (Wind)
Favor nutritious, warm, sweet, oily—and to a somewhat lesser degree—also salty and sour foods, as well as warm and calm behavior patterns. For example:
- Nutritious in this context means rich in protein and vitamins, etc.
- Sesame oil (internally and externally)
- Meat soup (if possible, cook with marrow)
- Lamb or mutton
- Raw sugar, molasses
- Rock candy

- Honey
- Nutmeg
- Saffron
- Licorice
- *Ghee* (clarified butter)
- Butter
- Garlic butter (moderate amounts)
- Butter with nutmeg (can also be used to massage reflex points)
- Cold-pressed seed oils
- Garlic
- Onion
- A glass of wine or beer on occasion doesn't hurt
- Favor all foods from regions that tend to be warm and mild
- Stay in a warm, pleasant place
- Avoid glaring lights
- Pleasant company promotes serenity
- Frequently take warm baths
- Allow yourself an oil massage now and then
- Sleep on a regular basis (a midday nap is also very beneficial)

When There Is an Excess of *Tripa* (Bile)

Favor cool, sweet, bitter, and astringent types of tastes with a cool active power, as well as cooling and calming behavior patterns such as:

- Yogurt
- Whey, buttermilk
- Fresh butter (moderate)
- Cool spring water
- Meat from a goat
- Meat from game
- Beef
- Black tea (in moderation)
- Dandelion leaves as a spring course of treatment
- Fresh grain mush of roasted grain (such as barley)
- Raisins
- Camphor (externally and very moderately; only against feverish conditions!)

- Saffron
- Favor all foods from regions that tend to be cool
- Stay in a cool place (for example, somewhat windy and shady)
- Lay down once in a while and rest
- Cooling fragrances (such as lavender, lemon) support a feeling of well-being

When There Is an Excess of *Péken* (Phlegm)

Favor hot, sour, and astringent types of tastes with coarse, light, and hot active powers, as well as the corresponding behavior patterns. For example:

- Pomegranate (above all, the seeds)
- Hot water
- Honey (above all, white honey)
- Ginger
- Coriander
- Black pepper
- (Greater and smaller) cardamon
- Cinnamon
- Black cumin
- Sea salt (in moderation!)
- Sea buckthorn
- Basically observe all of the advice for the "Activation of the Digestive Heat"
- Mutton or lamb
- Fish
- Stored grain (at least one year old)
- Grain dumplings from stored grain
- Seminola
- Favor all foods from dry, hot regions
- Occasionally drink a little glass of a ripened alcoholic beverage (such as hard liquor that has been aged for a long time)
- Only eat grains that have been roasted and cooked
- Stay in warm and dry places
- Wear enough warm clothing
- Do physical exercises every day
- Don't take a midday nap!

For Combination Types

In general, you can also influence combinations of the bodily energies in a beneficial manner through the above dietary and behavior patterns. In doing so, pay attention to your basic constitution and then attempt to determine the imbalance or excess of bodily energy (or energies) by looking at the symptoms, for example. A secondary excess of a second bodily energy may also exist under certain circumstances. By using the charts on the seasons, symptoms, and so forth, you can make your own evaluation. You can additionally intensify the effect by using the information about the distribution of the energies during the different times of the day. The following recommendations are very helpful for relieving the respective diseases:

Excess combination of	Relief through
Lung + Tripa	Cool and nourishing factors
Péken + Tripa	Cool and light factors
Lung + Péken	Warm and nourishing factors
Lung + Tripa + Péken	Cool, nourishing, and light factors

If you suffer from complaints in one individual organ, the following additional substances are recommended:

Organ	Substance
Heart	Nutmeg
Lungs	Bamboo concrement (inner pulp of the bamboo tree, which is difficult to obtain in the West); possible substitutes are calcite ash or the mineral kaolin (white clay).
Liver	Saffron
Kidneys	Smaller cardamom
Life channel	Clove
Spleen	Greater cardamom
Stomach	Pomegranate/(long) pepper

Additional Therapy Procedures

As already mentioned above, these additional therapy procedures—except for the gentle massage—should only be employed by people skilled in giving these types of treatments. Tibetan medicine includes the following additional therapy procedures:

- Oil therapies
    1. Internal
    2. External (massages, punctual applications)
- Moxabustion and therapy with the "Golden Needle"
- Moist fomentation, embrocation, hydrotherapy (such as baths)
- Humoral procedures of evacuation
    1. Enemas, suppositories
    2. Laxatives
    3. Emetics
    4. Cleansing of the channels
- Venesection (bloodletting)
- Cauterization (a burning therapy)
- Acupuncture
- Therapy with the copper vase (cupping)
- Therapy with the spoon (smaller surgery)

Oil Therapies

Both internal and external oil therapies are used in Tibetan medicine. The inner oil therapies are cleansing measures, the course of which may last up to three days.

These procedures are usually employed as preparation for enemas (see page 205f.), for rejuvenation treatments, and for the so-called "process of essence-extraction" (see page 229f.).

Internal Oil Therapy

The internal oil therapies can be done both orally and rectally. As a good possibility, the drinking of warm *ghee* is recommended for the oral form. (*ghee* = clarified butter; *ghee* is created by slowly boiling unsalted butter. The foam that comes to the surface is skimmed off, and the lower portion forms the essence or *ghee*. This process can be repeated several times to intensify the purification process. Another method of making *ghee* is very slowly boiling the butter without skimming off the foam that is produced, which is then boiled along with the butter. *Ghee* can also be stored outside of the refrigerator.) *Ghee* can also be inserted into the anus in suppository form. This measure serves to keep the mucous membranes in the intestinal tract smooth since an enema with water has a strongly drying effect on the mucosa. These accompanying measures of inner oil therapy are also very beneficial with the colonic hydrotherapy that is frequently used in the West.

Contraindications for inner oil therapy are greatly reduced digestive power, an imbalance of the bodily energy *Péken* (phlegm), gout, rheumatism, vomiting, and diarrhea.

External Oil Therapy

The external oil therapy is a form of *massage*. It is generally applicable when the corresponding indications are observed and the massage is basically done in a gentle manner. In Tibetan medicine, there are both techniques of massaging the individual pressure points or body areas in a "dry" way (such as the deep vibrational massage in the abdominal cavity to activate the organs), as well as techniques that use oil, ointments, and the like. Since the dry massage therapy employs highly specific techniques—with the danger of side effects when done improperly—the scope of this book will only discuss the specific points of the massage with oil pastes and ointments.

Punctual Application

Punctual applications are usually limited to small areas and are used for very specific symptoms. For each respective disease, a different ointment basis and various contents are selected. For example, an ointment of goat fat with hairy yellow oxtongue (*onosmodium*) is recommended against pustules in the face. When rubbed into the soles of the feet, an ointment of lard with caraway can be helpful against eye diseases.

In general, an ointment on the basis of buttermilk with soot and berberis mixed into it, among other things, is used against pimples and other skin ailments. An ointment to relieve gout is prepared as follows: black and white sesame seeds are ground and then boiled in rainwater (meaning water that is very fresh and rich in energy). This mixture should slowly boil until it becomes a paste. Some other recipes in Tibetan medicine, such as those against vitiligo (piebald skin), also include cow urine. An ointment of *ghee* or butter with nutmeg can be applied to the respective reflex zones when there is an excess of *Lung* (wind).

Oil Massages Against Disorders of the Bodily Energies

Oil massages, as described here, can be employed in most cases without hesitation. They serve both as preventive measures and means to activate the bodily powers of resistance, as well as gentle regeneration when there are slight imbalances of the bodily energies.

If you believe that you have falsely positioned vertebrae in the areas of the spinal column shown below, then have yourself treated professionally through gentle methods like osteopathy, rhythmic-energetic massages, manual therapy, acupuncture massages, Feldenkrais, and so forth. On a functional level, false positions of the vertebrae lead relatively frequently to imbalances of the bodily energies (and vice versa!).

Tibetan natural healing mainly uses the oil massages against diseases of the bodily energy *Lung* (wind). Massages are also recommended for older people to generally strengthen the body. A gentle massage of the entire body can be done for both of these general indications. Be sure you have a warm and pleasant massage environment with dimmed lights. The external setting, as well as the loving aura of the person giving the treatment, are very important criteria when there are *Lung* imbalances since stress exemplifies the cause *par excellence*. You can basically use any cold-pressed seed oil (except for mustard oil since it has a heating effect) for massage purposes. Warmed sesame oil is traditionally used in Tibetan medicine against *Lung* diseases.

If you would like to employ a somewhat more specific massage for the five subdivisions of the *Lung* energy, the body points and areas described in the following are advisable. The oil massage is employed for conditions like anemia ("pathological paleness"), for weak and emaciated people, against infertility, poor vision, and eating diseases. If one of the body areas depicted here is tender to the touch, this can be considered a sign of an imbalance of the *Lung* energy. In Tibetan medicine, the points are treated from top to bottom.

Massage of the *Lung* Points

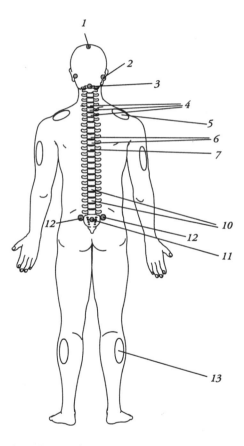

1 **Crown** = Gently rub in a few drops of warm sesame oil; highly recommended, especially for sleeplessness; corresponds with the pineal gland (epiphysis), the interface point between the spiritual sphere and the physical plane; massages on the crown mainly calm the "life-sustaining wind."

2 **Ears** = Gently rub in a few drops of warm sesame oil and possibly drip into ear; recommended against sleeplessness.

3 **Atlas** = First cervical vertebra (C1, C2): False positions can lead to *Lung* diseases; gentle massage on back of head can somewhat relieve the tensions; this vertebra corresponds with the pineal gland and the pituitary gland, among other things, and is therefore very important for the overall nervous and hormonal system.

4 **"Secret Wind Points"** = Gentle (!) massage one fingerwidth to the left and right of the fifth, sixth, and seventh cervical vertebrae. The seven cervical vertebra stands out clearly, so it can hardly be confused with the others; generally recommended when there is a *Lung* diseases; the points directly on the spinal column should only be used for diagnostic purposes; this area is connected with the thyroid gland and the parathyroid gland.

5 **Back of the neck and outer area of upper arms** = Gentle massages are very relieving for *Lung* diseases.

6 **Fourth and fifth thoracic vertebrae** (Th 4-5) = Points that are tender to the touch are frequently found one fingerwidth to the left and right of these when there is a *Lung* disease; these can be gently massaged; very important points for *Lung* disease! When a *Lung* disease arises during fasting, then first examine these points, followed by the sixth thoracic vertebra.

7 **Sixth Thoracic Vertebra** (Th 6) = This vertebra corresponds with the heart; the description of the spinal column under "Sternum" therefore basically applies to it as well.

8 **Sternum** = (Front side); extremely sensitive area that should only be treated by stroking it very gently (a very important *Lung* point: even touching this point gently can lead to crying and the like!); corresponds with the heart, the seat of the most subtle *Lung* energy, as well as the thymus gland, an important organ of the immune system. (For the position of points 8 and 9, see illustration on page 196; no. 4 + 5.)

9 **Solar plexus** = (Front side); this very important area of the body lies directly below the sternum; use gentle circular clockwise motions with the entire hand.

10 **Lumbar region** = The lower back primarily corresponds with the kidneys, which are particularly susceptible to cold diseases; it is therefore beneficial to generally keep this area of the body warm

and massage it gently; the massage should be done outward from the spinal column and, in conclusion, in a downward direction; in Tibetan medicine, the first and third lumbar vertebrae (= L1 + L3) are used for diagnosis and therapy; the adrenal glands are also effected by this.

11 **Sacrum, coccyx** = Points for *Lung* diseases are also found here (such as the "Gateway of the Wind," a point for the downward-voiding wind;) do warming, gentle strokes; sometimes just placing a warm hand on it is enough! In Tantric literature, these spots are considered "secret places." They are related to the reproductive glands.

12 **Sacrum-ilium joint** = This little, taut joint is considered the seat of *Lung*; these two joints can be perceived as dimples to the left and right of the sacrum; the so-called ilio-sacral joint plays a decisive role for the statics of the entire spinal column.

13 **Calf area** = Above all, when there is a chronic imbalance of the *Lung* energy.

As we can very clearly see from the areas mentioned above, the most important points connected with *Lung* diseases correspond with the endocrine or hormonal system. We can therefore assume that there is a very close connection between the bodily energy *Lung* (wind) and this very important body system. Furthermore, the conformity with the system of the chakras ("wheels of life") is obvious.

Special points for Tripa imbalances

- First thoracic vertebra = (Th 1): Considered to be the general point for the location and therapy of an imbalance of the bodily energy *Tripa* (bile).
- Seventh and eighth thoracic vertebrae = (Th 7-8): Corresponds with the liver and gallbladder; diseases of these organs manifest themselves as tenderness to the touch on the left and right side of these vertebrae and can also be treated here;
- Ninth thoracic vertebra = (Th 9): Together with the eighth thoracic vertebra, corresponds specifically with the gallbladder.

Special points for Péken imbalances

- The middle of the hands and feet are considered general points for the bodily energies *Péken* (phlegm). They are also connected to the *Lung* energy.
- Second thoracic vertebra = General point for *Péken* diseases.

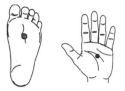

Further General Massage Points

Many of the points of Tibetan massage specified in the literature coincide with the meridian points of Chinese acupuncture theory. As previously mentioned, the indications differ, partly because of deviations in the way these two perspectives view certain energetic or anatomic correlations.

The massage points are very easy to find—if there is an energetic disease, the corresponding body point will be tender when touched! However, it isn't always very easy to differentiate between a painful point has too much or too little energy and/or with which of the three bodily principles this point is connected.

In general terms, an energy-rich point tends to create a bulge; a point lacking energy tends to create an indentation. Since the massage also activates or pacifies the bodily energies connected with the points, it is quite possible for imbalances and pain to be caused by improper treatment.

When massaging the neck and head area, it is advisable to first very cautiously feel the area and then also massage it gently. The Tibetan type of massage and pressure therapy done in the abdominal area should basically not be done by laypersons. But for the sake of general diagnostic clarification, be aware of possible changes in relation to the bodily energies: When there is an excess of *Lung* (wind), the belly will tend to be hard, bloated, and inflated; when there is an excess of *Tripa* (bile), the belly will tend to look sunken; people with a *Péken* (phlegm) disease will "carry around" a swollen and fat-filled belly.

In his book on *Kum Nye Relaxation*, Tarthang Thulku gives very precise information on self-massage, as well as auto-relaxation according to an ancient Tibetan system that he has further developed in a very wonderful way for the present age.

Massage represents a form of treatment that is highly valued by many people. There are also very few people who cannot give a massage. If you pay attention to your intuition, then the inner wisdom of your body will very precisely show you where and how it would like to be massaged. This can be very beneficial for alleviating lesser imbalances of the bodily energies.

Moxabustion and Therapy with the "Golden Needle"

These two procedures of the accessory therapies are both heat treatments. This means that they are primarily employed in connection with cold diseases caused by *Péken* (phlegm)and *Lung* (wind). Below is a general chart depicting the relationships of the spinal column with the bodily energies and the inner organs.

The points specified can be used for both diagnostic (sensitivity to pressure, bulges, indentations, swelling, blocks, etc.) and therapeutic purposes (when massaging, 1 1/2 fingerwidths next to the spinal column; for moxa, directly on the spine of the vertebra and possibly also next to the vertebra). Incidentally, the numbering of the vertebrae begins at the seventh cervical vertebra in the Tibetan system, but it has been adapted to the Western teachings about anatomy in the following lists.

Points and Zones of the Spinal Column

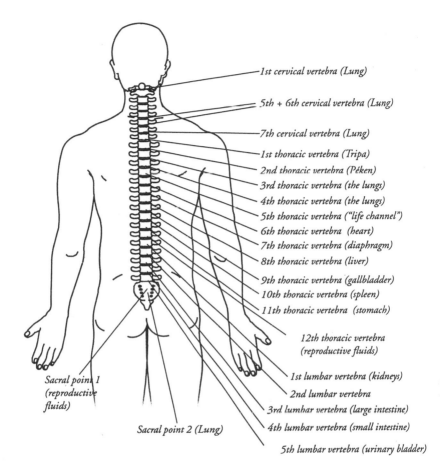

1st cervical vertebra (Lung)

5th + 6th cervical vertebra (Lung)

7th cervical vertebra (Lung)

1st thoracic vertebra (Tripa)

2nd thoracic vertebra (Péken)

3rd thoracic vertebra (the lungs)

4th thoracic vertebra (the lungs)

5th thoracic vertebra ("life channel")

6th thoracic vertebra (heart)

7th thoracic vertebra (diaphragm)

8th thoracic vertebra (liver)

9th thoracic vertebra (gallbladder)

10th thoracic vertebra (spleen)

11th thoracic vertebra (stomach)

12th thoracic vertebra (reproductive fluids)

1st lumbar vertebra (kidneys)

2nd lumbar vertebra

3rd lumbar vertebra (large intestine)

4th lumbar vertebra (small intestine)

5th lumbar vertebra (urinary bladder)

Sacral point 1 (reproductive fluids)

Sacral point 2 (Lung)

Cervical vertebra

- 1st cervical vertebra = Atlas = *Lung* imbalances
- 5th and 6th cervical vertebrae = General for *Lung* imbalances
- 7th cervical vertebra = general for *Lung* imbalances (for example, weakened memory, deafness, shivering; stiff neck)

Thoracic vertebra

1st thoracic vertebra = General against *Tripa* imbalances (*Tripa* diseases because of *Lung* and/or cold)

2nd thoracic vertebra = General against *Péken* imbalances (cold *Péken* diseases; pain of the respiratory tract; pain in the heart; possible increase of *Péken* and *Tripa* energy)

3rd and 4th thoracic vertebra = Upper and lower portion of the lungs (also points on the inner edge of the shoulder blade; diseases of the lungs and certain eye diseases)

5th thoracic vertebra = "Life channel" (general *Lung* energy; racing heart; heart diseases; weakened memory, loss of memory; intense sleepiness; delirium; combined *Péken/Lung* imbalances)

6th thoracic vertebra = Heart (indications as under "life channel")

7th thoracic vertebra = Diaphragm (for example, blocked diaphragm; if necessary, treat together with next vertebra)

8th thoracic vertebra = Liver (general liver diseases; vomiting; acute pain in liver area; excess of *Lung* and *Péken* in the liver, etc.)

9th thoracic vertebra = Gallbladder (digestive diseases, gallstones, lack of appetite, decreased digestive heat; constant headaches)

10th thoracic vertebra = Spleen (among other things, lack of drive; constant need for sleep)

11th thoracic vertebra = Stomach (decrease in digestive heat; gastritis; ulceration; diarrhea; general for stomach diseases)

12th thoracic vertebra = "Reservoir of the reproductive fluids" (among other things, uterine tumors, general abdominal diseases, diarrhea, intestinal diseases, spermatorrhea with blood)

Lumbar vertebrae

1st lumbar vertebra = Kidneys (cold diseases of the kidneys; cramps and pain in abdomen, etc.)

2nd lumbar vertebra = General point for hollow and full organs (general for cold *Lung* imbalances; general for diseases below the navel; general for diseases of the gallbladder)

3rd lumbar vertebra = Large intestine (general for large intestine; inflammations of the sexual organs; hemorrhoids, etc.)

4th lumbar vertebra = Small intestine (inflammations and general complaints related to small intestine; diarrhea; ulceration)

5th lumbar vertebra = Urinary bladder (bladder stones; increased frequency of urination; oliguria; cold knees, etc.)

1st sacral point = Reproductive fluids (prostate, uterus, etc.;
spermatorrhea; stiffness and paralysis of lower limbs, etc.)
2nd sacral point (center of sacrum) = "Gateway of the Wind" for
the downward-voiding wind (constipation, flatulence, diarrhea,
etc.)

The Practice of Moxabustion

In moxabustion (also called "moxibustion" or simply "moxa"), herb
cones of mugwort are either burned directly on the skin of certain
reflex points or indirectly through a needle or the like. Some herb
cones are also based on other heating herbs like nutmeg.

Energy is supplied to these specially selected reflex points when
they are heated. When the practitioner additionally uses a relatively
thick needle, of which at least the front section is made of pure gold,
this is called the *therapy with the "golden needle."*

This additional external therapy procedure is mainly employed
in the area of the anterior fontanel on the head. Among other things,
activation of the uppermost chakra is achieved in this manner. Many
mental diseases, such as depression or melancholy, are the medical
indications for this point.

Moreover, this is the point through which low blood pressure,
sensations of dizziness, dullness of the sensory organs, and hemiple-
gia—above all, imbalances related to *Lung* (wind) and *Péken*
(phlegm)—are treated. The therapy with the golden needle is frequently used before all of the other accessory "hot" therapies (such
as moxa, cupping, hot salt fomentation) since it shows very good
initial effects and therefore sometimes makes other accessory forms
of therapy unnecessary.

In contrast to this form of therapy, moxabustion can also be
performed on all of the points known to acupuncture. In the treatises of Tibetan medicine related to this topic, 71 specific moxa points
are used, of which 20 are on the front of the trunk, 22 on the spinal
column and rear section of the trunk, and 29 are on the arms and
legs.

According to another treatise ("King of the Moon"), considerably more points exist for the treatment with moxa therapy. In earlier times, Tibetan physicians sometimes had the mugwort cones

burn directly on the skin. The reason for this was creating extreme stimulation for the body through the regeneration of this artificial wound so that the immunological process would be effectively triggered. The moxa therapy employed in the West by naturopathic practitioners is certainly somewhat gentler. However, even in the West, the energetic principles of *Lung* (wind), *Tripa* (bile), and *Péken* (phlegm) must also be observed as the basis of this treatment.

According to the rules of Tibetan medicine, the mugwort used for the moxa treatment should be gathered in a clean place by a pure child in white clothing during the waxing moon under the supervision of a physician. Then it is dried and formed into cones. The size of the cone varies according to the choice of points. All moxa points located on or next to the spinal column are treated by applying a mugwort cone with the thickness of an index finger (at the basis of the cone).

For all of the other points, the basis of the cone corresponds with the thickness of the little finger. During the so-called "bloodletting," a moxa may be burned afterwards at the same point in order to cleanse the channels. This moxa has a flat form and the "size of sheep dropping." Moxabustion is generally used about six times. However, considerably more treatments may also be necessary over a longer time period in chronic cases.

Moxa treatments can be used for most cold diseases. The list of indications for them mostly includes *Lung* and *Péken* imbalances, as well as many diseases of the channels (arteries, veins, nerves, etc.), weak digestive heat, tumors, muscular tensions, anemic conditions ("pathological paleness"), and all chronic diseases.

In addition, the moxa treatments are applied in cases of mental diseases such as epilepsy or certain forms of mental diseases, the formation of nodes, and edemas. This treatment form should never be done directly on the sensory organs (such as the eyes or ears). Other contraindications are all conditions of excessive *Tripa* (bile) or diseases of the blood. Extreme caution is required when treating the perineum (the point between the anus and the testicles or vagina); some texts also proclaim a contraindication here. This point belongs to the so-called "existence vessel." This is the carrier of the reproductive fluids, and improper treatment at this point could trigger infertility.

Almost all moxa points can theoretically serve as pressure points for reflex zone massages. Above all, the four following points or body zones have traditionally been treated with moxabustion:

Traditional Moxa Treatment Points

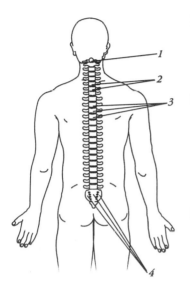

1. Back of the head in the area of the atlas (= first cervical vertebra), as well as to the left and right of it

2. Cervical spine in the area of the sixth/sevenths cervical vertebra (as well as 1 1/2 fingerwidths to the left and right of it, if necessary)

3. Thoracic spine in the area of the third/fourth/fifth thoracic vertebra (as well 1 1/2 fingerwidths to the left and right of it, if necessary)

4. In the area of the sacrum (on the so-called "Gateway of the Wind" at the center of the sacrum, as well as the so-called ilio-sacral joints to the left and right of the sacrum, which can be visibly perceived as little dimples)

Furthermore, all of the spinal column points listed under "Massage" (see *Oil Therapies* on page 179f.) can be used. While massage tends to be done next to the spinal column, the moxa treatment can also be performed directly on the spine of the vertebra (see above list of vertebrae, etc.).

The following moxa points are indicated for the head area

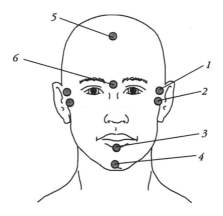

1 Toothache point = This point is exactly at the place where the ear is connected with the head. It is frequently used together with the point described on the ring finger (see page 198)

2 Important ear point (noise in the ears such as tinnitus, deafness, toothache, facial paralysis) = This point lies exactly at the center in front of the ear; a second point is located about one finger-width lower

3 Point for *Lung* (wind) imbalances (for example, memory loss) = This point is located at the center of the lower lip (lower edge)

4 Point for speech diseases, swelling of the tongue, etc. = This point is located exactly on the tip of the chin

5 Point for *Lung* and *Péken* disorders (such as poor eyesight) = The point is located exactly at the center of the forehead at the hairline

6 Point for nosebleeding, jaundice, etc. = The point is located exactly in the center between the eyebrows

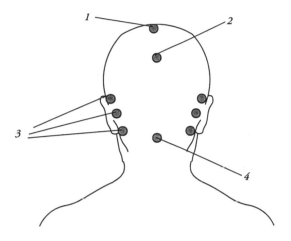

1 "Crown" = An important point for *Lung* disorders (see *Therapy with the "Golden Needle"*, page 186f.)

2 Anterior fontanel = A point for *Lung* disorders (such as dizziness, loss of consciousness, sleepless; also fever)

3 Three ear points between the ear and head = The upper two points are located directly on the crease between the ear and the head; the lowest point is located on the mastoid (= small bone about 0,2 inches) below where the ear is attached); all three points, but primarily the point on the mastoid, are treated for *Lung* disorders (noise in the ear such as tinnitus and other ear problems; complaints in the neck area; excessive talkativeness)

4 Occiput = At the base between the first cervical vertebra and the head (*Lung* disorders; nervous and hormonal system)

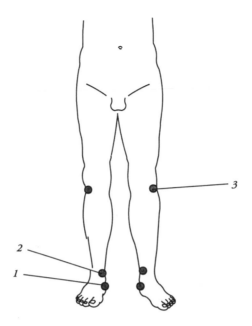

1 (In the distinct hollow) between the ankle and the heel bone, inner side = point for abdominal cramps, etc.
2 (In the distinct hollow) between the ankle and the tendon on the tibia (shinbone); inner side = point for impotence, etc.
3 On the little bone beneath the knee; outer side of the leg = point for stomach problems, etc.

General moxa points on the leg (back side)

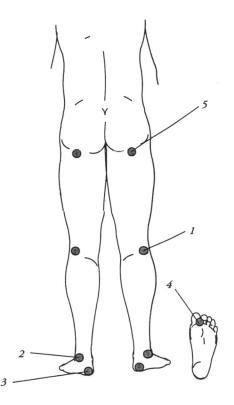

1 Thigh, outer side, in the hollow between outermost tendon and kneecap = Point for sensations of numbness, paralysis, etc., of the legs

2 Above the ankle, outer side (on the Achilles tendon) = Point for diseases of the pharynx (including speech difficulties)

3 Heel outer side, on the edge of the callosity = Point for eye inflammations, etc.

4 Large toe, inner side, at the joint cavity of the first joint (from the front) = Point for *Lung* disorders (for example, dullness of the sensory organs, depression, psychosis), hardening in the region of the occiput (back of the head); swelling of the testicles, etc.

Incidentally, this point also corresponds with the back of the head in foot reflex-zone massage

5 Approximately in the center of the gluteal fold = This point is related to the sciatic nerve; treatment of the legs in general

Important general moxa and massage points (front side of trunk)

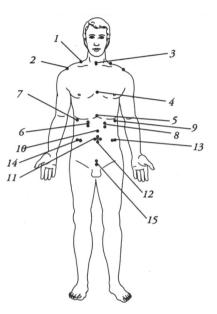

1 Point directly on the delta muscle (at the center, above) = pharynitis and tonsillitis, among other things; local point for shoulder stiffness

2 Shoulder height, at start of delta muscle, on the outside/above = General *Lung* point, for example: continuous nosebleeding, diseases in eye area

3 Exactly at the center of the upper edge of the sternum (fossa suprasternalis) = Important point for *Lung* disorders such as racing heart, spasms in heart area; tonsillitis

4 Center of sternum, exactly between the nipples = Important *Lung* point ("the boundary between black and white"); racing heart, loss of consciousness, depressions, etc.

5 Center, precisely below the xiphoid process of the sternum = Among other things, point for the stomach (general diseases, ulceration, etc.)

6 Approx. four fingerwidths from the center, right side below the costal arch and deeper = Two points for stomach and liver diseases

7 End of the free ribs, right side = General point for the liver

8 Approx. four fingerwidths from the center, left side below the costal arch and deeper = Two points for stomach and spleen diseases

9 End of the free ribs, left side = General point for the spleen

10 Approx. two to three fingerwidths above the navel, center = Point for the "Firelike Equalizing Wind" (important when there are digestive diseases)

11 Navel = Point for diseases in the abdomen in general; infertility, etc.; treat with extreme caution!

12 Four points around the navel = General points for the small intestine

13 Five to six fingerwidths to the left of the navel = Two general points for the descending portion of the large intestine

14 Five to six fingerwidths to the right of the navel = Two general points for the ascending portion of the large intestine

15 Approximately on the pubic hairline (and lower) = Points for the urinary bladder (retention of urine; anuria, etc.), prostate gland and uterus

General moxa points on the arm (back side)

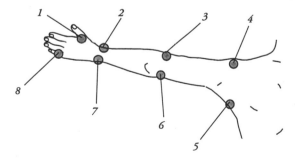

1 So-called "anatomical snuffbox" (visible dimpling) between thumb and index finger = Point for infectious diseases with fever ("contagious fever") and the related eye diseases

2 Little bone on the wrist (radial = pointing toward thumb), above = Disorders of the eyes, diseases of the brain, etc.

3 Little bone on the elbow (radial = pointing toward thumb), above = Point for local diseases

4 Shoulder height, start of delta muscle = General *Lung* point; for example, intense nosebleeding

5 On the axillary fold = General point for feeling of heaviness in upper half of body; general point for restricted movement of arm

6 Little bone on elbow (= olecranon; ulnary = pointing toward little finger) = Point for bone diseases

7 Little bone on wrist (ulnary = pointing toward little finger) = Point for skin diseases (such as warts)

8 On the metacarpophalangeal joint between the little finger and the ring finger = Point for diseases of the eyes; swelling inside the mouth, etc.

General moxa points on the arm (front side)

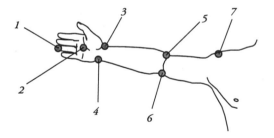

1 Tip of the ring finger and outer edge on the groove of the nail bed (ulnary = pointing toward the little finger) = Point for toothache (together with the ear points, see page 192)

2 Center of palm = General point for *Péken;* (also for *Lung*)

Additional points:

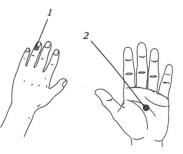

The other illustrated points correspond to the general points of the back side in the following way:

- Front side no. 3 corresponds with back side no. 2 (eyes/brain)
- Front side no. 4 corresponds with back side no. 7 (skin diseases)
- Front side no. 5 corresponds with back side no. 3 (elbows)
- Front side no. 6 corresponds with back side no. 6 (bone diseases)
- Front side no. 7 corresponds with back side no. 4 (*Lung* point)

Since moxa is a heat treatment, you should never drink cold water directly afterward—because water extinguishes fire! In addition, moxa should not be performed directly after a meal, and you should not have any opulent meals directly after a moxa treatment. Furthermore, on the day of the treatment you should avoid all sour and fermented foods (vinegar, lemons, yogurt, etc.), as well as all behavior patterns related to *Lung* (wind) and, above all, *Péken* (phlegm). In order to intensify the effect of moxa, a little walk or the like is recommended after the treatment.

The points of the moxa treatment, especially in the head and neck area, are also used for the **treatment with hot oil.** In this form of treatment, which is primarily used against *Lung* imbalances, a piece of material is dipped into hot oil. This is then dabbed onto the appropriate reflex points. In order to intensify its effect, the material can also be filled with herbs and the like.

Moist Fomentation, Embrocation, and Hydrotherapy

The external therapy forms of moist fomentation, embrocation, and hydrotherapy—which are also frequently employed in Western naturopathy—are generally used in Tibetan medicine when the bodily energies of *Péken* (phlegm) and *Lung* (wind) are imbalanced. They are also applied in cases of digestive diseases, abdominal cramps, and lymphostasis. One of the contraindications for hot fomentation, etc., is diseases of the bodily energy *Tripa* (bile); further general contraindications are related to anemic conditions based on a *Péken* imbalance, such as hepatitis. There are two forms of embrocation, warm and cold.

Cold Embrocation

Cold embrocation is generally applied in cases of hot diseases such as inflammations. Cold water that has been drawn from a fountain or spring is used for this purpose. Since Tibetan medicine is strongly oriented toward the cosmological factors, the water is drawn before sunrise in order to employ the cold energies of the night for therapeutic purposes. For some indications—such as colic of the small intestine—water that has been drawn by starlight is used. Many people in the West may make light of this cosmological approach, but the distinct intensification of the effect by including the corresponding natural force is a reality for every therapist who works with energy. After all, it is the detachment of the human being from the unity with the natural archetypal forces and entities that ultimately leads to illness. In the West, the only place that this concept of unity can still be found is within the alchemical-spagyric tradition, as well as its further development within anthroposophic-oriented medicine.

A living example of this particular tradition can be seen in so-called "Easter water": according to tradition, this is drawn from a spring on Easter Sunday at sunrise. This water has a very intense curative effect and can be stored for one year without spoiling. The Tibetan tradition describes the "natural water with the eight qualities." In addition to rainwater, which always has these qualities, water that is drawn whenever the "Rishi star is shining in the heavens" has them as well. This astronomic point in time is always between the end of August and the end of September.

Now back to Tibetan medicine: For application purposes, the cold water is either put onto the body in the appropriate containers (such as animal intestines) or poured directly onto it. The latter is a form of hydrotherapy. Soluble powders of medicinal plants or minerals are frequently mixed into the water. For example, white aconite with lotus bark is recommended as an additive for the above-mentioned colic of the small intestine. A cool loam pack, which is placed between the eyes or behind the neck, is recommended against nosebleeding. To relieve inflammations, for example, cold river gravel is placed on the corresponding areas of the body.

Warm Embrocation

The warm embrocation, as well as the use of moist warmth and *baths* (= hydrotherapy) is employed for both old and cold diseases. The Tibetans are very imaginative in their choice of medicinal substances to be used for this purpose. For example, coagulated blood in the liver is treated with an embrocation of warmed moss that has had dried grain mixed in with it.

River gravel is also heated and applied in the case of clotted blood because of a traumatic incident (such as a blow). Digestive diseases of the stomach are treated with an embrocation of heated pigeon droppings, and wearing furs around the kidney area generally relieves coldness of the kidneys. A fomentation of salt that has been wrapped and heated in towels is recommended for general digestive diseases with flatulence and so forth, as well as abdominal colic.

Muscle tension, nodules in the musculature (myogelosis), stiffness, lameness, and general diseases of the bodily energy *Lung* (wind) offer a general area of application for moist warmth and baths. Wherever it is possible, hot springs are used for this purpose. Hot springs are seen as the most effective form of baths. They very frequently have distinctly effective natural mineral components, which are selected accordingly to intensify the effect. When there are no hot springs available, hot baths with the addition of the appropriate minerals and plant decoctions should be employed. A mixture of mugwort and soda, for example, is suggested as a remedy against lameness of the limbs and old wounds. There are many remedies included in the *Materia Medica* that can basically be used in this manner.

Venesection (Bloodletting)

The accessory therapy form of "bloodletting" is related to the idea of venesection in the naturopathy of the West since the intention is to extract "the bad" blood (meaning blood permeated with contagious materials). The essential difference is that in Tibetan medicine usually just a few drops of blood are caused to flow out at precisely defined body points. Many of these points coincide with the moxa points or the points for the smaller surgery (see "Therapy with the Spoon").

The actual operation occurs with a lancet or a similar pointed and sharp instrument. The method of bloodletting is only used when the disease cannot be healed through the measures of medication and/or cannot be collected in its own location. As a preparatory measure for Tibetan venesection, the patient is given a decoction of various myrobalan fruits or of myrobalan fruits with long pepper, alant, and the like to drink for one to three days. This serves to separate the "healthy" from the "diseased" blood.

If this measure cannot be accomplished, at least a general warming of the body should occur. In addition, the operation must immediately be stopped as soon as the "diseased" blood stops flowing and the "good" blood begins to flow out since this could otherwise weaken the life essence. Bloodletting is never performed at places where the various channels flow together and never where the so-called *La* (= the vital essence, see *Non-Visible Forces,* page 79f.) is located at the present moment.

The suitable indications for bloodletting are mainly diseases of the bodily energy *Tripa* (bile). In addition, diseases of the blood, swelling, lymph diseases, tumors, wounds, and gout, as well as certain types of fever, are considered appropriate illnesses for venesection.

It is inappropriate to perform venesection on people who are weak and old, children under 16 years of age, all patients with *Lung* diseases, as well as pregnant women or women who have just given birth. Venesection is also inadvisable after the administration of other drastic measures such as enemas, emetics, etc.

As a follow-up treatment, either massage or moxa with mugwort in the form of small, flat little cones (shaped "like sheep droppings") is used at the puncture point. This is done to cleanse the channels, as well as to soothe and distribute the strongly occurring

Lung in this area. The only exception to this is the throat area. After venesection, refrain from all types of factors that stimulate the bodily energies *Tripa* and *Lung*. This means do not drink any alcohol, do not become too warm, etc. In order to pacify the accumulating "wind," drink a bone-marrow broth or eat some honey, for example. Be sure to rest after such measures have been taken.

Without going into detail about the indications of the individual body points, at least the possible coloration of the blood for differentiating between imbalances in the bodily energies should be mentioned here. In a *Lung* imbalance, the blood will show a dark color with reddish-yellow foam and have a "coarse" consistency. A *Tripa* imbalance manifests itself in yellowish blood and/or a purulent smell. A *Péken* imbalance is revealed as a light red, thick, soft blood. In all of these cases, bloodletting is usually only used once. Incidentally, healthy blood has the color of vermilion.

Cauterization

This form of external accessory therapy, which may seem rather archaic to the Western individual, is performed with a hot cautery.

Cauterization represents a further intensification of the accessory therapy procedure since this drastic technique is only done after a longer treatment period with pills, etc., or in difficult cases. The cautery is available in many different sizes, but they all should have a gold-plated copper tip.

This therapy is also a form of heat therapy, which means that it is primarily used in cold diseases of *Lung* (wind) and *Péken* (phlegm). Its rules and points are similar to those mentioned for the massage (see *Oil Therapies,* page 179f.) and moxabustion (see page 186f.). The *Lung* points on the back of the head and the upper spinal column appear to be the main candidates for cauterization. If the cauterization needs to be intensified, the appropriate herb is placed on the respective area of the skin, such as bamboo silicate on the joints or juniperus (a type of cypress) against cold diseases.

Incidentally, the gypsies, who, as we know, originated in India, also use cauterization. However, it appears that they employ different—and probably fewer—points. During the 1950s, the French physician Nogier observed that the gypsies in his region frequently had "burned" (= cauterized) points in their ears. In answer to his questions, they told him that this was a way of treating acute sciatica. Nogier was so enthusiastic that he began to examine the ear systematically as a reflex zone for the entire body—and this was the birth of modern ear acupuncture!

Acupuncture

Acupuncture has mainly become known in the West through Traditional Chinese Medicine. Since this is a mild, yet invasive method, it appears to not possess the same high ranking in Tibetan medicine as it does in the Chinese medicine.

Yet, there is an independent form of Tibetan acupuncture. Among other things, the choice of points is different from the Chinese practice since certain energetic and/or anatomical correlations are viewed and interpreted differently by both schools of medicine. Moreover, the Chinese perspective of the energy paths (meridians) does not necessarily serve as the basis for the Tibetan type of acupuncture. Since this topic may not be of interest to the general reader, it will not be discussed in detail within the scope of this book.

Humoral Procedures of Evacuation

When an excessively strong accumulation of bodily energy occurring during its own specific season cannot be pacified through the relieving measures of dietary and behavior patterns, medication, etc., the accessory therapy forms of evacuation measures are used. Among these evacuation procedures are:
- Enemas (or suppositories) for an imbalance of the bodily energy *Lung* (wind)
- Laxatives for an imbalance of the bodily energy *Tripa* (bile)
- Emetics for an imbalance of the bodily energy *Péken* (phlegm)
- Cleansing of the channels

These cleansing procedures work according to the principle of removing the excessive bodily energy that has accumulated during the season of its manifestation through the closest body opening. This pacifies the imbalance in order to reestablish harmony within the bodily energies. Moreover, these therapies can be used in order to eliminate possible remnants of old diseases from the body.

Elimination of *Lung* (wind)

An excess of the bodily energy *Lung* (wind) mainly accumulates during the summer and can be eliminated from the location of the large intestine during its time of manifestation—autumn—through an *enema* or *suppositories*.

Tibetan medicine differentiates between the mild and the drastic forms of enemas. While the mild forms of clyster and enema are used for the slighter intestinal diseases and microorganisms in the intestines, as well as against cold diseases of the kidneys or lower back area and inner *Lung* tumors of the intestines, the more drastic forms of the enema are employed against such problems as major disorders of the "downward-driving wind," intense constipation, retention of urine, certain infectious diseases, fresh tumors, and so forth. Substances such as sodium hydrogen carbonate, stitchwort, garlic, Spanish fly (*Cantharis*), and the like are applied.

The inner and, if necessary, external oil therapy serves as a preparatory measure. The inner oil therapy keeps the mucous membranes supple since the enema with water dries out the intestinal mucosa and causes even greater imbalances as a result. Enemas are not appropriate for the following conditions: edemas, *Péken* disorders, certain liver diseases, as well as certain states of fever.

There are at least one dozen different recipes for *mild enemas* listed in Tibetan medicine. Many of them are related to specific illnesses. In case of a slight excess of the bodily energy *Lung* (wind), a suppository made of a piece of ripened butter that is at least one year old can be used as the basic remedy. A mixture of water with *ghee* and/or milk and/or boiled mutton broth can be used as the basic liquid for all enemas. These light forms of treatment are frequently adequate for pacifying an excess of *Lung* energy.

If only the bodily energy *Lung* is disturbed, then powdered juniper, long pepper, rock salt, and *Myrobalan chebula* can be added to this basic liquid. If an imbalance exists that is a combination of *Lung* and *Tripa*, the basic liquid is a broth from animals that live in damp places (such as fish, duck, and goose), which is added in place of the mutton broth. If an imbalance exists that is a combination of *Lung* and *Tripa*, the basic liquid is made from the broth of animals that live on dry land (such as beef, goat, chicken) instead of the mutton broth. Varying the basic recipe is a simple, yet effective method of application. Many recipes with animal components can also have plant recipes substituted for them without diminishing the effectiveness.

Elimination of *Tripa* (Bile)

An excess of the bodily energy *Tripa* (bile) primarily occurs during the late summer or early autumn. Above all, it becomes stored in the area of the small intestine. **Laxatives** are administered for purification purposes.

Additional indications for this accessory therapy are certain types of fever, anemic conditions, edemas, lymphostasis, rheumatism, and certain types of poisoning. This therapy is discouraged in the following cases: people who are aged or too young, in the winter, during pregnancy, in the case of *Lung* diseases, as well as when there is foreign matter in the intestinal region. As applies to all evacutive measures, a preparation phase is also employed in order to ripen the illness. The appropriate washing and massage corresponds approximately to the preparation phase described under "*Péken*" in the following section.

The laxatives are divided into mild and strong purgatives, whereby the respective specific medicinal ingredients for the corresponding disease are mixed into the appropriate basic remedy. The basic mixture generally consists of rock salt, various types of rhubarb, long pepper, knotgrass, and *Myrobalan chebula*. Examples of further substances that are employed are madder, wolf's-milk, wild lettuce, purging cassia, castor oil seeds, and the like. In addition, Tibetan physicians use additional herb pills or decoctions, if necessary. In individual cases, this depends on the type of disease and the specific constitution of the patient.

Elimination of *Péken* (Phlegm)

Since an excess of the bodily energy *Péken* (phlegm) is usually formed during the winter and stored mainly in the stomach, it can be eliminated at the time of its manifestation, meaning spring, through the appropriate medication of *emetics* (vomitives).

Since *Péken* generally tends to sink downward, without a purifying procedure this would otherwise have a negative effect on the digestive heat. Basic indications for emetics are considered poor digestive power, gastritis, ulceration, poisoning, acute abdominal cramps, as well as certain diseases in the head area. This form of treatment should not be used in the case of most *Lung* diseases or for very young or very old individuals.

A preparation phase is necessary here as well. This aims to cause the illness to ripen at its location. This phase may take several days and is supported with the appropriate medicinal remedies. This preparation phase can be "shortened" by washing the entire body with a decoction of mugwort.

According to tradition, fermented grain is also mixed in with this remedy. Afterward, the person is massaged with a cold-pressed oil such as sesame oil. This measure should be performed in the evening, and the patient should go to bed when it has been completed. The next morning, the actual emetic is administered. For this purpose, there is also a basic mixture of calamus root, rock salt, long pepper, thistle, mustard seed, and wolf's-milk. The decoction of these substances makes a relatively mild emetic. On the other hand, the dried and powdered substances create a more drastic emetic. The appropriate medicinal substances can be added to this basic combination according to the respective mixture ratio between the imbalance of the bodily energies.

The entire process of evacuating the bowels or vomiting is very intensive and definitely exhausting. Tibetan medicine urgently advises against using these applications without the help of a qualified practitioner.

If a Tibetan physician does not succeed in eliminating the disease from the body by using these measures, the accessory method of **"cleansing of the channels"** can be employed. This is the last remedy of choice in this series of eliminatory procedures. After the appropriate preparation phase, the patient receives a decoction of cayenne pepper and mallow to inflate the channels. Afterward, a very clearly established procedure for the actual cleansing of the channels occurs, whereby various powders and pills with the main component of Spanish fly are administered.

Therapy with the Copper Vase
(Cupping)

Cupping is a procedure that is also frequently used in Western naturopathy. After the respective areas of the body have had creme applied to them, a fire is lit beneath a container (made of glass in the West, a copper cup in Tibet) in order to create a vacuum. The container is then quickly placed on the appropriate area of the body and sucks upward an area of the skin with the size of the cupping container. This results in an intense skin arching—with the corresponding stimulation.

Cupping is usually performed on the reflex points of the inner organs in the trunk area of the body or on places where there is an intense accumulation of toxins (for example, on the delta muscle of the neck). This form of dry cupping is employed for cold conditions that frequently manifest themselves through a so-called "retraction" of the body tissue. The so-called "wet cupping" is also used in the West for extracting "impure" blood, which has toxins in it. This area has fine needles or the like stuck into it beforehand. An ointment can be applied afterwards to intensify the effect on the body area treated in this manner. This method must obviously be performed in a clean manner. The indications in Tibetan medicine and in Western naturopathy (in the sense of humoral pathology) appear to hardly differ from each other.

Therapy with the Spoon
(Smaller Surgery)

This represents the most drastic of all therapy forms in Tibetan medicine, which is only applied as the very last possible approach. As is also common in Western medicine, for example, punctures are mainly performed for the purpose of draining pus, serum (lymph), and so forth.

The total of 110 body points for puncturing, curettage (scrape), and further smaller surgeries are essentially the same as those for moxabustion. However, there are naturally further points that result from the respective location of a node, tumor, swelling, cut, or a broken bone. In the 22nd chapter of the *Explanatory Tantra*, the surgical instruments for treating the above-described cases are shown. However, a detailed discussion of them is beyond the scope of this book.

In earlier times, it appears that surgery was a field practiced with success in Tibetan medicine. However, the performance of larger surgeries was stopped after a death in the royal family that occurred during such an operation. The Tibetan perspective that every surgery represents a drastic intervention and therefore should only be practiced as the end point of all therapeutic efforts must be underlined.

Each operation ultimately represents a defeat for the therapy of the self-regulating healing powers of the organism. This approach should therefore only be used as the very last possibility. Western medicine has achieved extraordinary technical progress in this area, which—especially in emergency situations—appears to be a clear advantage. However, the all too frequent use of surgery (including transplant surgery) is not the ultimate answer.

Perhaps some diseases should truly be viewed and accepted within the larger context and also from the perspective of karma.

In Tibetan medicine, patients suffering from an illness that will probably end in death are instructed about the appropriate spiritual possibilities. A lama will enlighten the patient as to the suitable prayers and mantras, in addition to healing actions, as well as providing spiritual support.

These prayers and actions—such as freeing an animal that was intended to be slaughtered, the ritual of circumambulating the stupas, and the like are meant to create a positive level of resonance for the patient so that he or she can take leave of this physical plane in a peaceful manner. This creates an outstanding starting position for a good transition into the worlds of the intermediate state (*Bardo*) between this life and the next. The hospice movement in recent years has placed wonderful accents in this direction and offers the dying person a dignified departure from this world.

The Medicines

General Comments about Collecting and Mixing Medicinal Substances

The enormous variety of substances used in Tibetan medicine is quite impressive. It includes all areas of life—the mineral kingdom, plant kingdom, and animal kingdom. By these means, the various levels of human existence are invited to heal in a holistic manner. Some human substances are described in the medical treatise. However, these are generally not employed. Many of the animal substances are also no longer used today. It is the minerals, including the gemstones and metals, and the plants that represent the overriding portion of the medical substances that are used today. Mixing them in a well-balanced manner into an overall composition of many components is a highly scientific, yet intuitive art. The ability of Tibetan remedies to initiate a synergistic-complex healing effect without any simultaneous undesired secondary reactions has often been praised.

Tibetan pharmacology is a mystery in itself and can never be learned without the help of a physician who is skilled in it. Although many recipes are easily accessible, it is practically impossible to make a remedy only on the basis of this information. This would involve enormous difficulties. The terms employed have changed in the course of the centuries, and some plants may already be extinct. Synonyms are also frequently used for certain substances—some of the substances named after animals are really plant parts with the corresponding appearance. Abbreviations used only in certain regions create additional confusion.

Up to now, not very much literature has been available in Western languages about the *Materia Medica* of Tibetan medicine. An excellent source of this is, for example, Dr. Pasang Yontens Arya's *Dictionary of Tibetan Materia Medica*. A further, very easily accessible source is Dr. Barry Clark's translation of *The Quintessence Tantras of Tibetan Medicine*, which also contains a large portion of the *Materia Medica*. Dr. Clark is one of the few individuals of Western origin who has succeeded in first learning the Tibetan language, then thoroughly studying Tibetan medicine in its theoretical and practical aspects, and then specifically working through the *Materia Medica*. His courses, which take place on a regular basis, can be recommended to anyone who is interested in Tibetan medicine. The *Materia Medica* by Dr. Arya also symbolizes a great enrichment of the literature available in English. Courses held by Dr. Arya take place on a regular basis in Italy, and Germany. For more information see *Selected Bibliography* on page 239f.

The information on the weight of each individual substance in a recipe is usually given within a very relative framework since a description like "one handful" can be interpreted in different ways. Without the help of a physician skilled in pharmacology, it is not possible to make one single mixed remedy. Not too long ago, Tibetan physicians also made their own remedies. Because of the well-known situation in Tibet, as well as a basic lack of personnel and funds, the medicinal remedies are mainly produced today by the Tibetan Medical Institute in Dharamsala. In order to preserve this aspect of human cultural heritage, more distinct efforts—especially in the field of remedy mixtures—would be necessary on the part of the West. This would be especially helpful in the form of financial and technical assistance. It would be very tragic if this immense knowledge was lost forever.

Tibetan Remedies in the West

It is relatively difficult to find physicians for Tibetan medicine to consult in the West. Although some of them travel in Western countries on a regular basis, the number of physicians who have a permanent practice in one place can be counted on one hand. In addition to the woman physician Dr. Nel de Jong (Amsterdam, The Netherlands) and Dr. Pasang Yonten Arya (Milan, Italy), there are two more Tibetan clinics in The Netherlands that have permanently employed physicians working at them. Tibetan physicians also practice in Switzerland, like Dr. Dönckie Emchi, Great Britain, New Zealand, and North America (for more information see *Addresses* on page 240.) In addition to difficulties in finding a physician, the possibilities of procuring the remedies are also quite complicated.

One of the Tibetan types of remedies that is relatively easy to obtain is the preparation *Padma Basic*. In the practice, it has proven to be very effective in treatment of the corresponding indications such as circulatory diseases, chronic hepatitis, and so forth. There are many studies on this preparation that are oriented on the Western scientific study criteria such as the randomized double-blind trials. However, here as well, the diagnosis must be the first step in any course of therapy.

Another possibility for strengthening yourself with Tibetan recipes are the healing teas mixed from herbs and spices from the appropriate sources. Western palates usually need to get used to the taste of his teas. There are currently four different tea mixtures with very clear application possibilities available.

For more information see *Addresses* on page 240.

The first *tea mixture* was created to be a general purification and detoxification tea for harmonizing and regulating the metabolism. This means that it can be enjoyed daily as a type of "house tea." As a tea break, this tea contributes to a general harmonizing and energizing in the middle of a hectic day. There certainly is truth to the Eastern saying that a leisurely cup of tea serves inner collection and promotes mental harmony—an important precondition for health itself! The next tea mixture was made especially for the accompanying symptoms of the monthly cycle, as well as for menopausal complaints, and is certainly a relief and a comfort for women. Because of its composition of aromatic herbs and spices, the third healing tea promotes the warming of the entire body and is formulated especially for the cold days of winter. Its corresponding contents—such as rose hip, ginger, various types of cumin and pepper, cinnamon, and so forth, serves to strengthen the body's immune system.

Good digestion is one of the keys to health. A corresponding tea has been mixed for the digestive diseases that occur so frequently in modern civilized societies. This mixture has a stimulating effect on the entire digestive system and promotes better absorption of the nutrients after a meal, for example. Above all, the contents stimulate the functions of appetite and digestion, which are roused by substances like pomegranate seeds, ginger, galangal, cardamon, various types of pepper, or wormwood.

In addition to the general dietary and behavior patterns, tea mixtures are a possibility for each of us to personally influence ourselves according to the principles of Tibetan healing. Various Tibetan herb teas can also be ordered. For more information see *Addresses* on page 240.

Collecting and Processing the Herbs

Tibetan herbs are traditionally gathered during different seasons of the year. This is always started by a pure child dressed in white and accompanied by a physician. The mantra of the Medicine Buddha or a similar beneficent mantra is recited. The times for collecting are generally determined in the following manner:

- Stalks, stems, and certain roots are gathered in autumn, when the fruits have already dried.
- Leaves, certain resins, and fresh plants (such as sprouts) are gathered during the summer rainy season when the plants are fully ripe.
- Blossoms and fruits are gathered during the autumn winds, when the fruits are ripe.
- Bark, resin, and roots are gathered in spring, during the growth phase.

Moreover, the exact time of gathering is determined by the calculation of the auspicious planetary days during the general period of the waxing moon's second week. Only undamaged substances from a clean environment should be collected. Furthermore, the "rule of correspondence" (= active power through equivalents) applies to both gathering and mixing. This means that substances with warm or hot active powers are collected in the valleys that face south and/or in deeper areas—the warmer parts of the country—and herbs with cooling active powers can be found in valleys and slopes that face north and/or higher, cooler locations.

This rule of correspondence, which correlates with our Western "theory of signature," is a determining principle—together with the principle of tastes and post-digestive tastes—in the use and mixing of Tibetan medicinal substances. For example, a bean with the form of a kidney (*Canavalia gladiata*) has a positive effect on the kidneys attributed to it, and the kidney of an animal is also said to have the corresponding effect on a human kidney. However, animal components are practically no longer employed. Because its external appearance is similar to that of a brain, the mineral halloysite has a positive effect on the human brain attributed to it. The velvety cowage (*Mucuna entada*) is considered to be helpful for the spleen, the yellow plum (*Choreospondia axillaris*) for the heart, and the fruit of the entada tree (*Entada phaseoloides*) for the liver. This principle of "active power through congruity" primarily became known in the West through Paracelsus.

After gathering, the plants and plant parts are cleaned. If possible, water from the same region should be used for this purpose. Then they are broken into small pieces with wooden sticks in such a way that part of the plant juice flows out. This form of processing probably breaks open the cell structure of the plant, simultaneously creating a type of "seal." It results in better possibilities for using the contents. In any case, simply drying the plants without this procedure is considered to be very harmful for the contents in Tibetan medicine. The principles of the signature theory are also followed during the drying process. This means that cooling plants are dried in the shade and warming plants are dried in the sun or with heat. The general rule is that dried plants can be stored for up to one year without losing too much of their effective components.

Compounding of Medicine/
The Medicine Buddha

The actual compounding of the substances into a medicinal composition in the form of powders or pills occurs in a contemplative manner. This includes pure thoughts, visualization of the Medicine Buddha, as well as recitation of the Medicine Buddha mantra.

The physician imagines that the Medicine Buddha appears in the space in front of him or her. He is blue in color and sits cross-legged in the lotus position on a lotus blossom. The left hand rests in his lap and holds a bowl filled with *Amrita*, the essence of all nectars. His right hand is in front of his right knee, with its palm facing the observer. A uniquely enchanting flower—the "Magnificent Victorious Myrobalan" is growing out of his right palm. This plant always appears as the blessing of a Buddha visiting the earth. It possesses all six tastes and heals any cold or hot diseases. The Medicine Buddha radiates multicolored light from his heart center. The observer—in this case, the Tibetan physician who is compounding the remedies—is completely permeated by this light and cleansed of all diseases of the three mental poisons. As much as possible, this mental attitude is maintained during the entire compounding process and supported by reciting the Medicine Buddha mantra. In its brief form, here is this mantra in its Tibetan form:

"Tayatha om bekentzé, bekentzé maha bekentzé—
radza samudgate soha!"
(Tibetan)

"Tadyata Om bhaisajye bhaisajye mahabhaisajye raja
samudgate svaha!"
(Sanskrit)

"OM! Honor to grace, to healing, to the highest healing—
King of healers! So be it!"

During the recitation, the remedy is transformed into pure nectar, and all suffering and misery is eliminated when a person takes this remedy. People with the corresponding initiation turn into the Medicine Buddha themselves during this meditation.

This visualization is also very helpful during the treatment of patients, which is why Tibetan physicians frequently use it. If you are not a Buddhist, you can visualize any healing energy, such as Christ, in a similar form with multicolored light. This purifies both the remedy and the patient with whom you may be working at the moment. It also clearly shows that the actual healing impulse always comes "from a higher place" and the physician is only the mediator of this energy. A clear channel will naturally also be able to convey a clear healing energy.

As the "highest physician and healer," the *Medicine Buddha* has a long tradition with various names. In Sanskrit, he is called *Bhaisajye*

215

Guru, among other things. The Tibetans call him *Sangye Menla.* This is why there are also different mantras.

There is also a bit of disagreement among scholars about the exact blue coloration of the Medicine Buddha. According to Dr. Arya and Dr. Clark, the Sanskrit word *vaidurya* (pronounced *baidurya*) means a very clear and valuable gemstone. So they both classify it as "aquamarine." However, other scholars and translators call *vaidurya* "glass" or "beryl"; even more frequently, it is also labeled "lapis lazuli."

An idea for harmonizing the most frequently named approaches of "aquamarine" and "lapis lazuli" comes from my companion, Heidi Mayrock, who conveys her work in archetypal cosmology with beautiful images. According to her, the idea of the aquamarine is like the light blue of a radiantly sunny day; on the other hand, the dark of the lapis lazuli with all of its gold traces is like looking into the star-filled sea of the nighttime sky. These are the two sides of the same Buddha light.

Selected Substances of Tibetan Medicine

The substances discussed here should under no circumstances be used without the assistance of someone who is very knowledgeable about them. In Tibetan medicine, one individual substance is practically never taken alone. In addition to the desired effect on a specific organ or a specific bodily energy, an individual substance almost always also has a certain negative side effect. In order to guarantee the optimal and harmonious effect, a remedy is usually created from at least three to four substances. Up to several dozen different substances are mixed into the differentiated compositions (there are medicines with over one-hundred active ingredients!). The complex effect of these medicines is not produced in the sense of a scattershot therapy, but rather in a synergistic way where there is a balancing order that optimally supports the effectiveness. The "composing" of this type of remedy is a high art.

Please be aware that some of the substances listed here are toxic in their non-detoxified form. When used improperly, all substances can become poisonous. Even presumably "harmless" medicinal plants should not be used for longer than two to three weeks at a stretch in the form of tea or the like since "the amount makes the poison." Only after a break—sometimes longer, sometimes shorter—can the respective tea then be used as a beverage again.

Metals

All metals basically possess a distinctly high ranking in Tibetan medicine. Above all, a variety of different metals (such as purified mercury) are made into the so-called "jewel pills," a Tibetan medicinal specialty with the general indications of detoxification, long life, energy, and powers of resistance. They are also administered against paralysis, epilepsy, brain diseases, and various forms of tumors. For all metals, both the various areas of origin and the related special qualities are usually described. The following section is intended to provide a small selection of metals with their respective taste and post-digestive taste, as well as an insight into the possibilities of their medicinal applications.

Gold is described in a variety of colors and has an astringent taste, an astringent post-digestive taste, and cooling active powers. Gold is generally considered to be a life-prolonging strengthening remedy, an antidote for various forms of poisoning, and is also used to drive away spirits. Gold ore, from which gold can be extracted by smelting, is administered for diseases of the lymph.

Silver is described as having an astringent taste and post-digestive taste. It is thought to have drying properties. As a result, it is considered for diseases related to the lymph, pus, or blood. Similar to gold ore, silver ore is used against lymphostasis and the like.

Copper has a sweet taste and post-digestive taste, as well as a cooling active power. Copper also has a drying effect and is applied, for example, against heat diseases of the liver and the lungs.

Iron has a sour taste and cool active powers. Among other things, it is used against certain swellings, as well as diseases of the liver and eyes.

Iron ores: Hematite has a sour and astringent taste and drying effect. It is used for diseases of the liver, the bones (such as broken bones), and the brain. It has an extractive effect on the lymph fluid. *Magnetite* has a similar application spectrum as hematite, but is also used to expel metallic foreign bodies from the intestinal tract. *Meteoric iron* is used to regenerate nerves.

Red lead is employed against such conditions as necrotic states (decay processes in the cell tissue).

Tin and tin ore promote the growth of the musculature.

Zinc is used against eye diseases and to promote the regeneration of wounds. In addition, it prevents excessive sweating.

Mercury represents in its purified form an indispensable component of the "precious jewel pills". Because of its constant mobility, it is ascribed to the mental aggregate and the bodily energy *Lung* (wind). In its normal form, mercury is a deadly poison—but in its purified form, it is an outstanding healing remedy. In this quality as well, it is very similar to the mind, which is only "whole" in its purified form. Among other things, purified mercury is used for prolonging life, as a general tonic, and as a detoxification agent.

Gemstones

All pure gemstones possess the utmost healing qualities. The worse the quality of a gemstone, the less healing qualities it has. The Master of Medicine, the Completely Awakened One, the Highest Healer, sits on a of completely pure gemstones. His clear light radiates in all directions in order to ease the torment of all the unfortunate and woeful states of existence. The diamond (Sanskrit *vajra*, Tibetan *dorje*) is considered the indestructible primeval energy of the universe. However, this must also be understood in the figurative sense.

In the *Root Tantra*, the gemstones of human beings are attributed with the inherent quality of easing all suffering caused by poisons, spirits, (mental) darkness, swelling, and fever. In addition, the light of the gemstone is considered capable of "cleansing everything." Furthermore, gemstones of human beings are capable of fulfilling wishes.

Moreover, the gemstones of the gods (*devas*) have additional qualities. Among other things, they are completely pure and can speak. The gemstones of the Bodhisattvas (enlightened beings who enter into the world of appearances because of compassion in order to show all suffering beings the path of liberation) have such additional qualities as being able to give teachings. Through them, the Bodhisattvas have the possibility to recognize the time of absolute liberation for other beings.

In the following section, some of the gemstones used in medicinal mixtures are described.

Turquoise is used against liver poisoning, heat diseases of the liver, and fever caused by poisoning.

Lapis lazuli is used against leprosy, poisoning, and diseases of the lymph.

Malachite relieves the "harm from the twenty-eight constellations of the moving stars." One of these types of harm is epilepsy. Malachite is employed for diseases of male sexuality and also for drying out the lymph fluid. It is also known to be a hair restorer.

The following precious substances can also be included in this list:

Pearl and *mother-of-pearl* are used against poisoning and are also extremely beneficial for the brain. However, in Tibetan medicine the word "pearl" means not only the types of pearls that grow in oysters and clams but also the bright red pearl from the brain of a certain type of snake or a bright blue pearl from southern India that is found in trees after the rain. There is also a "pearl" in the peacock, which is used especially in the case of poisoning.

Red and black *coral* is used against various types of fever (such as fever of the liver). The coral is also employed for fever based on poisoning.

Pyrite is considered beneficial against eye diseases, as well as against rabies. In addition, it appears to have a favorable influence on diseases of the brain such as obsession, as well as against lymphatic diseases. The pyrite inclusions in lapis are used in the combination effect with it.

The *gzi stone* (chalcedony/agate) is considered to be a stone that is holy and brings protection. It has "eyes," meaning black circles, and is said to come from the time when the land that is now Tibet was still on the floor of the ocean. Among other things, it is used against poisoning, fever in the bones, and eye diseases.

The shell of the large **sea snail**, among other things, is divided into the superior (clockwise) and inferior (counterclockwise) type in terms of its spirals. It is pulverized and applied against diseases of the eyes and bones and accumulations of pus. Certain types of mussels also have a similar effect.

Other Minerals

Carbonate of lime is mixed into remedies against diseases of the bones, the ligaments, and the tendons. Calcite is considered an important remedy for rejuvenation elixirs.

Coal dissolves gallstones and kidney stones.

Talc cleanses the channels and is helpful with stones.

Saltpeter is also applied for the dissolution of all types of stones and relieves urine retention. The old form of producing "saltpeter" was to burn green barley. It is used for the cleansing of tumors and generally for increasing bodily warmth.

Potash is used to increase the general heat, meaning the ripening of certain processes.

Natron serves to eliminate undigested grain, as well as being an antidote for poisoning.

Yellow sulfur is used against diseases caused by spirits and it has a drying effect on pus and lymph. Black sulfur is employed against certain skin diseases such as erysipelas.

Plants

The main components of each medicinal mixture are all the parts of plants from the roots to the flowers. The gathering and drying of plants was described in previous sections. Here is a small selection of the plants that also grow in the West. Some of the plants listed below propagate in many subspecies, which are sometimes identified in different ways by the various authors. For the purpose of simplification, only the general (family) name is given for these plants. For example: In the Tibetan *Materia Medica*, at least six different subspecies of "larkspur" are mentioned. Here only the family name of *Delphinium* is used. On the other hand, the exact plant name is used in the distinct identification. For example, *Paeonia veitchii* is used for the peony or *Gallium aparine* for a type of bedstraw.

Within this context, it should be mentioned once again that Tibetan medicine almost never treats diseases with just one individual substance. Instead, through the mixture with additional substances it always ensures that possibly occurring imbalances of the bodily energies and/or side effects are relieved or do not occur at all. Some of the plants mentioned here are very toxic (such as aconite, henbane, hemp, etc.) These plants in particular should never be used without the cooperation and help of a practitioner skilled in herbal therapy. As already mentioned, even the presumably "harmless" plants produce highly active substances.

The Highest of All Plants

Unfortunately, the "Magnificent Victorious *Myrobalan Tree* (*Arunamgyal*), which is considered the *highest of all healing plants*, only grows during the times of a Buddha. It possesses all six tastes, as well as the three post-digestive tastes, all eight active powers, and the twenty characteristics of illness. In Tibetan medicine, this type of myrobalan is considered to be like a "wish-fulfilling jewel." However, we can also make use of the three other types of myrobalan. Although these do not possess all six of the tastes, some do have up to five of them. The fruits are usually used, but the bark and middle layer of the bark are also employed sometimes.

Kabul myrobalan/panicled myrobalan tree (*myrobalan chebulia* = *terminalia chebula; arura*) is comparable to a large walnut tree in terms of its bark and has all of the tastes except salty. This tree is the universal remedy of Tibetan medicine. It is considered extraordinarily nourishing, longevity promoting, and sparks the digestive heat. In terms of its fruit, there are up to eight subspecies with correspondingly different areas of application such as eye diseases, demonic possession, digestive diseases, the healing of wounds, bile diseases, etc.

The other types of myrobalan basically have similar healing effects:

Myrobalan bellerica (= *Terminalia bellerica; Barura*) can be used when there are imbalances of *Lung* (wind), *Tripa* (bile), and *Péken* (phlegm). Lymph diseases are also one of its indications.

Myrobalan emblica (= *Emblica officinalis; Kjurua*) is also employed against imbalances of all three bodily energies.

Additional Plants

Larkspur (*Delphinium*) is bitter tasting, has a cooling active power, and is helpful against infestation with lice and heat conditions of the bile, such as those that manifest as diarrhea. One type of *delphinium* is also employed against insect bites and poisoning, as well as for driving away spirits. Generally, the blossoms are used.

Cress (Lepidium) is somewhat hot and bitter in taste. It is used to dry up excess lymph in the chest area, as well as applied against lymphostasis in general. In addition, cress is beneficial for the bones.

Gentian (Gentiana) grows in a great variety of forms. The taste of gentian is generally bitter; its active power is coarse and cooling. It is usually employed against an excess of *Tripa* (bile) or *Lung* (wind). Red gentian is used against various types of fever, jaundice, and hepatitis, as well as generally against an excess of *Tripa* (bile). The white type is used against inflammations, among other things. Gentian cures fever in the hollow organs, is effective against inflammations of the gall bladder, and has a distinctly detoxifying effect. Black gentian is also used against inflammations of the hollow organs. Furthermore, some people have an allergic reaction to the bitter constituents.

Iris (Iris) is biting-hot and bitter in taste with sweet and sour post-digestive taste, as well as a cooling active power. The blossoms are used, as well as the seeds, which have a heating active power. Iris is used against an excess of *Lung* (wind), as well as against diseases of the blood and fever. Some types of irises are considered helpful against intestinal worms, as well as being a general laxative. They increase the body heat, neutralize poisons, and relieve cramps. They are pain-relieving and beneficial against diseases of the eyes and ears (such as tinnitis).

Hemp (Cannabis sativa/indica) is used against diseases of the lymph, skin diseases (such as pimples, itching, etc.), and diarrhea, as well as eye diseases. Hemp pacifies *Lung* (wind) and is considered an aphrodisiac. It has a sweet and astringent taste, as well as a mild active power. Hemp is subject to the Dangerous Drugs Act.

The blossoms of the ***willow tree*** *(Salix sp.)* are used against chronic fever conditions and swellings that form around wounds. Cases of poisoning and the swelling that they cause can also be treated with willow (i.e. the bark).

Various portions of the *elm* (*Ulmus*) can be used to rub into the joints (arthrosis, arthritis). Similar to the willow, it also has a beneficial effect on swellings that form around wounds.

Various portions of the *poplar tree* (*Populus sp.*) are also applied for healing wounds. The poplar has indications similar to those of the willow.

The root of the *ginseng* plant (*Panax ginseng/Pseudoginseng*) is a general strengthening agent. Ginseng collects and binds toxins and eliminates them from the body. In addition, it is considered to be an agent against intestinal worms. It is also used for strengthening in times of general epidemics (such as the flu), as well as against fever. The taste of ginseng is bitter and astringent.

Cranesbill (Geranium) is used against various types of fever, such as fever accompanying the flu. Its taste is sweet and biting-hot, with oily and cool active powers. An additional beneficial effect against diseases of the eyes (such as cataracts), intestinal worms, pneumonia, and swelling of the limbs is ascribed to cranesbill. Primarily the roots are used.

Wild rose (such as *Rosa sericea, Rosa sertata,* and *Rosa omeiensis*) is used by Tibetan medicine to collect and bind toxins in the body. In addition, it is beneficial against diseases of the lymph, for healthy tooth growth, and against imbalances of the bodily energy *Lung* (wind). Wild rose blossoms mitigate the bodily energy *Tripa* (bile). Complaints caused by "non-visible forces" can also be relieved by it. The *rose hip* (from *Rosa sericea*, for example) is added to the mixture for imbalances of the bodily energies *Tripa* and *Lung* and used against fevers caused by poisoning or heat of the liver. It has a sweet, as well as a sour taste and an oily active power.

The *castor-oil plant* (*Ricinus communis*) serves as a laxative and emetic, mainly when there is an excess of the bodily energy *Péken* (phlegm). Castor-oil seeds are considered to be a drastic type of laxative. The taste of castor oil is bitingly-hot, bitter, and sweet. Its active power is heating.

Acorns (from the various types of *Quercus*) are used in a pulverized form to end diarrhea.

Longwort (*Angelica archangelica*) is hot, bitter, and sweet in taste. It is used against cold diseases of *Lung* (wind) and *Péken* (phlegm), such as diseases of the kidneys, stomach, heart, swellings, distention, poisoning, and lymph diseases. It is also employed for inflammations of the ears, infectious diseases, epidemics, leprosy, and uncontrollable bleeding. External fomentation is also prepared from this extraordinary healing plant.

Five-finger (*Potentilla*) has a somewhat bitter taste. Some say that it drives away all the spirits with its sweet fragrance. It is used as an emetic, against poisoning, and for healing wounds.

Veronica (*Veronica*) has a bitter taste and cool active power. It is used against feverish conditions based on poisoning, against acute states of pain, and against infectious diseases. Its penetrating smell drives away non-visible forces.

Mugwort (*Artemisia*) has a hot and bitter taste. This is an extraordinarily versatile medicinal plant; for example, the annual mugwort is used against diseases of the lungs and pharyngitis. Other types of mugwort are considered beneficial against kidney disease, swellings, and various *Tripa* diseases. Certain types of mugwort have rejuvenating qualities ascribed to them. Mugwort is also made into moxa cones.

Mallow (*Malva verticillata*, among others) has a sweet and astringent taste and produces heat. It is used against diarrhea and kidney diseases, swellings, etc. Mainly the seeds of the mallow are used.

Aconite (*Aconitum*) is considered an extremely potent and simultaneously highly toxic medicinal plant. Most types are bitter or biting-hot in taste and have a cooling active power. They are used against fever, pain, enteritis (inflammation of the bowels), and poisoning (by snakes or scorpions, among other things), as well as generally when the bodily energy *Tripa* (bile) is imbalanced.

Thornapple (*Datura stramonium*) is a very toxic plant. It has a bitter and biting-hot taste, as well as cooling active power. Its seeds are used to cure wounds, swellings, infections, toothaches, and pain conditions in general. The thornapple is also considered to be an aphrodisiac.

Henbane (*Hyoscyamus niger*) is also very toxic and is considered to be an antidote against intestinal worms and tumors, among other things. Disorders of the lungs and toothaches are among the indications for this plant remedy. Henbane is said to strengthen the sex drive (= aphrodisiac). The seeds are the part of the plant that is used. Its taste is bitter and biting-hot with neutral active power.

Wild strawberry (Fragaria) can be found in almost every forest. It has a somewhat sweet taste with cooling and coarse active powers. Its effect is styptic and drying. It is used for *Lung* disorders of the large intestine. An additional area of application is in the form of an emetic for diseases in the upper part of the body (especially the lungs), as well as diseases of the blood.

Wild blackberry (Rubus) can also be found abundantly in most forests. However, in Tibetan medicine the inner layer of the bark is mostly used. The taste is sweet and sour, and the active power is astringent and heating. The blackberry is beneficial against imbalances of the bodily energy *Lung* (wind), various forms of fever, diseases of the urinary tract, weakness of the sensory organs, and coughing. It is considered a kidney tonic. Another type of blackberry is described as sweet and astringent in taste, as well as neutral in its active power. It is used against all inflamed diseases of the nasopharyngeal space, as well as the bronchial tubes (colds), and harmonizes the three bodily energies.

Valerian (Valeriana officinalis) is used against chronic fever conditions, poisoning with fever, as well as possession by spirits.

Dead nettle (Lamium) is used for healing wounds and edemas. The active power is mild. Other types of nettles can be used to promote digestion (especially of green vegetables). The *stinging nettle (Urtica)* creates heat and cures chronic *Lung* fever.

Forget-me-not (Myosotis) is used for drying pus accumulations, as well as for the treatment of wounds. The roots of the forget-me-not can be very helpful in cases of tooth decay.

Fenugreek (Trigonella foenum-graecum) is a medicinal plant that is also frequently used in Europe. It is mixed into remedies against diseases of the lungs and intestines (including diarrhea), infections, and fevers, as well as for the general healing of wounds since it possesses the ability of extracting pus. Fenugreek is also very beneficial for the spleen and stomach. It has a bitter taste with cool active power.

Maidenhair fern (Lepisorus) is used for healing wounds and against certain types of fever, among other things. It is also considered to be beneficial for the bone marrow. It is said to extract pus and relieve diseases of the gallbladder. Other types of ferns (such as *Corallodiscus*) are described as having a bitter and sweet taste. These ferns can neutralize toxins and favorably influence diseases of the reproductive organs, as well as those of the kidneys and bladder. They are also used for healing wounds. This type of fern can also be mixed in with remedies against diarrhea. The male fern (*Dryopteris*) is used in cases of excessive *Tripa-* energy, as well as against poisoning.

Parsley fern (*Tanacetum*) is used to stop bleeding, as well as against swelling of the limbs and kidney diseases. It also has rejuvenating effects ascribed to it.

Tagetes (*Tagetes*) has a sweet and bitter taste. It is used against pus in the lungs, as well as for healing wounds.

Pasqueflower (*Pulsatilla*) is hot and bitter in taste. It increases the digestive heat and has a favorable effect against lymphatic diseases and tumors. This plant is toxic.

The (white) *alpine rose* (*Rhododendron*) has rejuvenating qualities. It is used against disruptions of the *Péken*-energy. This plant is toxic.

Stonecrop (*Sedum/Rhodiola*) has sweet, bitter, and astringent taste with cool active power. It is considered beneficial for the lungs and can be applied as a mouthwash against bad breath. This plant is slightly toxic.

The *peony* (*Paeonia veitchii*) is mixed into remedies for the treatment of surgical erysipelas. The exact translation of its name would be "lotus root." This plant is slightly toxic.

Varieties of *clematis* (*Clematis*) are described as having a biting-hot and slightly sweet taste. Their active power is heating. Both the stem and the blossoms are used. The clematis increases the digestive heat and has a beneficial effect against tumors. The Tibetan clematis has yellow flowers and has a reputation for destroying "cold," meaning benign, tumors. This plant should be used with caution.

The various types of *aster* (such as *Aster flaccidus*) are bitter in taste, cooling in active power, and beneficial against poisoning and fever, such as the fever accompanying the flu. They have a styptic effect and are considered to be a general tonic. Imbalances of

Lung (wind) are the primary area of use. Some asters drive away spirits. The flower is the main part used as a medicinal substance.

Lousewort (*Pedicularis*) has a bitter and astringent taste, as well as cooling active power. The blossoms are used for irregularities of the "downward-voiding wind" in the area of the seminal vesicle and vagina. Lousewort is considered to have a detoxifying effect and be extremely healing for inflamed diseases of the liver and gallbladder, as well as for the gastrointestinal tract with diarrhea. Other varieties of pedicularis (such as P. *pyramidata*) are considered to be sweet and astringent in taste with heating active power, as well as being beneficial for both hair growth and the reproductive fluids.

Bedstraw (*Galium aparine*) is considered to be very beneficial against imbalance of the *Tripa*-energy, jaundice, and inflammations of the paranasal sinuses.

Knotgrass (*Polygonum*) has a sour, bitter, and astringent taste. Its active power is cooling. The root is usually employed for medicinal purposes. It is used against inflammations (= "fever") of the small intestine and large intestine, as well as hot diarrhea. Lymphatic swelling, chronic diseases, as well as diseases in the hip and pelvic area (such as kidney diseases) are also among the possibilities of application.

Sorrel (*Rumex acetosa*) frequently grows in meadows in their natural state. Its taste is sour. It can be applied against various forms of fever, as well as skin diseases and poisoning. Curled sorrel (*Rumex crispus*) is sweet and bitter with a cool post-digestive taste. It is used as a wound-healing agent and as a laxative.

Crowfoot (*Ranunculus*) has a hot-biting taste and a heat-creating effect, as well as a drying effect on swellings. In addition, it has a beneficial effect against tumors, increases the digestive heat, and fights putrefaction processes. Crowfoot also has a beneficial effect on injuries of the tendons. The flower is the part that is most frequently used. This plant is toxic.

Sage (*Salvia*) is slightly sweet and astringent in taste. It has a cool active power. It is very beneficial against diseases in the mouth-throat area (can be used in the form of rinses), as well as against eye diseases (used as a compress) and thirst. Moreover, sage has a healing effect on the stomach and an overheated liver.

Catmint (*Nepeta*) has a distinctly powerful smell, as well as a hot and astringent taste with cooling active powers. Among other things, it is applied for disinfecting wounds since it is considered beneficial against the invasion of microorganisms (such as in infections). Moreover, it is used against stomach cramps, as well as fever.

Plantain (*Plantago*) is considered beneficial against diarrhea, for healing wounds, and for extracting excessive lymph fluid. Plantain is helpful in cases of urine retention because it has an diuretic effect. Its taste is sweet and astringent, and its active power is cooling.

Shepherd's purse (*Capsella bursa-pastoris*) is applied against vomiting, among other ailments. It is good for the lungs and kidneys. Shepherd's purse has a sweet and hot taste.

The *pine* (*Pinus sp.*) has a hot taste, as well as dry and coarse active powers. It is used against cold diseases, meaning an imbalance of *Lung* (wind) and/or *Péken* (phlegm). Furthermore, it is said that the tree can dissolve tumors. Pine roots are used against various gynecological diseases. The ashes of the pine or fir tree are used against various venereal diseases. The resin of the pine is beneficial for the lymph fluid, above all in the head area, as well as for the bone marrow.

Camphor (*Cinnamomum camphora*) is extraordinarily cold and must be used with extreme caution. It is considered the "king of the cold remedies." Camphor is a very dynamic acting plant that can be used against very high and chronic, deep-rooted fever. Camphor has a bitter, hot, and astringent taste, as well as very cold, very coarse, light, and hard active powers.

Rejuvenation and the
Process of Essence-Extraction

The term "rejuvenation" is used in Tibetan medicine for all cleansing procedures that simultaneously contribute to the strengthening of fertility and the life force. This is why all remedies and behavior patterns with an aphrodisiac effect are discussed here.

In Tibetan medicine, all substances that accelerate the production of regenerative fluids and clearly improve their quantity and quality are understood to be aphrodisiacs.

Since the regenerative fluids represent the last essence in the chain of bodily constituents, they could even be called the essence of the essence on the physical level. The process of forming these essences lasts about six days. However, a substance with an aphrodisiac effect has the ability of accelerating this process so that it is completed within a few hours (even within one hour for some substances). But this does not mean that there will be an immediate gain of pleasure in the physical sense. Instead, there will be an extraordinary increase in the general physical and mental powers. This may be expressed in an increased ability of concentrattion and a clearer complexion. If this power is then further sublimated through meditation, it can result in extraordinary physical and mental progress. This procedure is called "the extraction of the essence" and is accompanied by the ingestion of the so-called "essence-extraction pills."

Any intake of physical food is stopped for a period of three, six, or twelve months. Instead, three essence pills are taken every day. Some yogis even considerably extend this amount of time. Dispensing with the intake of food has the advantage that the body receives only the pure essence of certain substances in the form of pills; and, it no longer must expend energy to digest normal foods.

The power of concentration can be considerably increased as a result. The related meditation practice is mainly described in the so-called *Six Yogas of Naropa*, a secret Tantric teaching of great strength and effectiveness. Since these teachings also contain certain dangers, they are only passed on from the experienced teacher to the qualified student by word of mouth.

The pills taken in the "extraction of the essence" consist of a great variety of blossoms for the most part. These flowers have been gathered, dried, and then pressed into pills according to the guidelines for collecting (see *General Comments about Collecting and Mixing Medicinal Substances,* page 210) with the appropriate cleansing, mantra recitation, etc. The flowers must be completely pure. As secondary constituents of the pills, blessed substances and substances for the respective imbalances may be added.

Cleansing Measures

Cleansing measures form an initial treatment for the long-lasting "process of essence-extraction." They are also used for chronic ailments, very deep-rooted diseases, and the like. In general, the cleansing measures usually also last several weeks. The diet is adapted to the patient's condition in keeping with strict rules, and the patient must also follow the corresponding behavior patterns.

The *external measures of cleaning* consist of such simple things as baths, oil massages, and subsequent rubbing with pea flour. Various substances, depending on the patient's illness, can be mixed in with the bath water. The *internal measures of cleaning* consist of inner oil therapy (see page 179). Sesame oil, *ghee*, and garlic butter are mainly used for this purpose. The garlic butter is made as a very strong mixture and contributes to avoiding the formation of excess *Lung* (wind); furthermore, it eliminates microorganisms and the like. Among other things, the ingested *ghee* keeps the mucosa supple and makes sure all *channels* (gastrointestinal tract, arteries and veins) are flexible. In addition, other cleansing measures like laxatives or enemas may be advisable, depending on the patient's condition. These remedies are also mixed with the respectively appropriate substances.

Tibetan medicine does not use *fasting* in the same form as propagated in the West. Only in the case of acute illness is the intake of any type of food stopped for one to three days, if necessary. But even then, at least hot water, meat broth, or rice broth is usually consumed. Fasting increases the bodily energy of *Lung* (wind) for a long time. People with this type of constitution should be very cautious about fasting. It is frequently more advisable to employ the so-called "*relief days*," upon which only certain forms of grain in roasted form or only steamed vegetables or rice mush with ginger or meat broth is eaten. When this is done, the bodily strength can generally be maintained over a long period of time and none of the bodily energies will be disturbed for long.

Selected Diseases and the Possibilities of Influencing Them Through Diet and Behavior

There are no clear "recipes" for the treatment of general diseases in Tibetan medicine since each of these can consist of very different combinations of imbalances of the individual bodily energies. However, less severe diseases can be influenced in a positive manner through general dietary and behavior patterns. The following advice is intended as general possibilities for strengthening the digestive or immune system, etc., and should not be understood as causal therapy. It is naturally also obvious that every supposedly "minor" disease could also have deeper causes and may require an expert naturopathic-medical clarification. Be attentive toward your bodily energies and react in a flexible manner. Nevertheless, one-fourth of all diseases in Tibetan medicine are classified as having such a slight nature that additional medical treatment can be dispensed with.

Pharyngitis (Throat Inflammation)
Pharyngitis can be influenced in an extremely favorable way by changing the behavior and dietary patterns. Since this is a hot condition, you should give preference to cooling and nourishing measures. Honey or molasses in warm milk is also beneficial. Decoctions of rose hip, ginger, anise, fennel, cardamom, and many other herbs and spices are advantageous for generally strengthening the immune system. If you want a more convenient solution, you can buy an immune-strengthening tea that has these herbs (in addition to many others) in a balanced mixture.

If there are *intense symptoms as a result of an influenza infection* or the like, you can fast for one to three days and just drink hot water. If you tend to have an excess of *Lung* (wind)or you are very weak, then also drink hot rice mush and meat broth or vegetable broth.

Fever

In Tibetan medicine, fever is differentiated into many different types with various causes and symptoms such as pain in the limbs, headache, lethargy, extreme dryness of the mouth and mucous membranes, etc. The common factor is a distinct overheating of the entire organism. Consequently, cooling measures should be preferred and heating measures avoided. Allow yourself rest, avoid any type of excessive physical strain, and do not expose yourself to the direct heat of the sun. Avoid strongly spiced foods and meat. Also abstain from alcohol and very heavy foods. Eat rice mush, whey or buttermilk and yogurt, and drink cool water.

Diarrhea

The main cause of diarrhea is a imbalances of the digestive activity. The digestive heat may either be too low, which indicates an excess of the bodily energy *Péken* (phlegm), or there is an excess of *Tripa* (bile). In any case, *Lung* (wind) is involved. When there is an excess of *Tripa* (bile), the cause of the diarrhea may also be an inflammation of the gallbladder or an overheated liver. In any case, you should additionally supply your body with minerals. One way of doing this is drinking salted water.

Absolutely avoid unhealthy substances like coffee, nicotine, or alcohol. It is basically true that every form of diarrhea is very beneficially influenced by fasting. If there is a secretion of mucous in the stools and you feel like you have "stones in your belly," you should have a meat soup or vegetable soup or a rice decoction. You can also add some salt, coriander, black pepper, ginger, and possibly some butter to the rice. Keep your abdominal area warm. In some cases, warm fomentation (wraps) around the belly and waist area are advantageous.

If the diarrhea is caused by an excess of *Lung* (wind), this can be recognized by the foam that forms on the surface. Warm and nourishing components, such as meat soup or vegetable soup, rice decoctions with butter, etc., are helpful here as well. You can also employ butter suppositories and oil massages. Diarrhea caused by an excess of *Tripa* (bile) has an extremely spontaneous character and quite an unpleasant smell. Eat roasted rice and avoid all sharp and hot spices and the like. You can also drink some buttermilk or whey.

Constipation

Constipation can also be caused by an excess of all three bodily energies. In any case, a drying of the intestinal tract has occurred. The cause of this is frequently a lack of exercise and/or weak musculature of the abdominal wall. If the constipation is caused by *Lung* (wind) or *Péken* (phlegm), the belly will be bloated. The stool will have the character of sheep droppings. In some cases, it will be difficult to get rid of the intestinal gas.

When the constipation is caused by an excess of *Tripa* (bile), there will frequently be pain in the abdominal area. The basic rule for all forms of constipation is: Exercise on a regular basis! Drink ample amounts of fluids (in the form of ginger decoctions when there is a *Péken* imbalance and cool water for *Tripa* imbalances.) Eat several light meals, such as steamed vegetables. Fresh fruit juices may also be helpful. Avoid bananas and chocolate, as well as fatty and heavy foods. You may also want to do some form of intestinal cleansing.

PadmaLax, a medication made by the firm Padma according to the Tibetan example, can also be used against constipation. In any case, it is important to follow the rule that, at latest after three days, a skilled practitioner should be consulted for clarification.

Sleep Disturbances

The most frequently observed forms of sleep imbalances are strongly related to the bodily energy *Lung* (wind). However, irregularities of the other two bodily energies may also play a role.

Your sleep behavior is a very clear reflection of your general state of health and, above all, the condition of your "nerves." Warm and pacifying measures (such as oil massages or light point massages on the roof of the skull and the 7th cervical vertebra, warm baths, rice, meat broth, honey, warm water, etc.) have proved to be beneficial.

A light walk before going to bed also serves to "decongest" the mental activities. Don't eat anything heavy, fatty, and raw in the evening. Instead, have soups and steamed vegetables. If you have no digestive diseases, a glass of warmed milk with honey can be helpful.

Lack of Appetite

If you suffer from a lack of appetite, you should reread the chapter on sparking the digestive heat (see page 102f.) since poor digestive heat is frequently the cause of this situation. Different sensations of taste may also accompany a lack of appetite. For example, food may taste very bitter when there is an excess of the bodily energy *Tripa* (bile).

A lack of appetite can also be related to a feeling of "being full"— both in the physical, as well as the emotional sense. A time of quiet and cleansing would be appropriate in this case. For inner cleansing, calamus, ginger, pepper, cardamom, coriander, honey, salt, molasses, and lemon can be used. The corresponding tea mixtures also have a very beneficial effect on the digestive performance. Buttermilk or whey are also considered helpful. In any case, a drink of ginger with honey is beneficial.

Heart Complaints

The treatment of tachycardia and nervous heart complaints can be favorably influenced through a gentle massage in the middle of the sternum, at the upper indentation of the sternum, as well as on the seventh cervical vertebra. A *Lung* disease is frequently the basis for this, which means that warming and pacifying measures are most important. Under some circumstances, the cause of this can also be discovered in the improperly functioning joints of the spinal column (for example, when the small intermediate joints are blocked).

Concluding Observations

We can all take responsibility for an important portion of our own preventive health care. By recognizing our own individual type of constitution and having a lifestyle that harmonizes with it, we can do a great deal in this direction.

Nutrition plays an important role in the life of every human being; it is therefore clear that the kitchen is where a change toward better health begins. Begin, for example, by stocking some of the herbs and spices mentioned in this book on your kitchen shelf.

Let increasingly more of your knowledge about the correlations between the elements, active powers, etc. flow into your daily food preparation. Drinking the appropriate decoctions is also a simple form of health care. When necessary, drinking the healing tea mixtures mentioned here also generally serves to promote good health.

Match your behavior patterns with your basic type and pay attention to your personal changes during the course of the seasons.

The diagnostic possibilities listed in this book, such as observing the morning urine, can give you important additional indications of what is happening within your body. Integrate the suggestions given there with care and steadfastness, but don't expect any premature results since only a certain continuity can bring healing. In its general application, Tibetan medicine is a wonderful gift for all human beings. For the specific treatment of a disease by a skilled Tibetan physician, it becomes a true blessing.

Short Test for Classifying the Personal Body Energy

For easier orientation, you can fill out both of the following short questionnaires. The first test will help you determine your constitution types, meaning your basic type classification. The second test will help you determine any possible imbalances of your bodily energies. For certain questions, multiple answers are possible: For example, a person can be in both a windy *and* a hot place at the same time, etc.

Give yourself:
3 points for very frequent occurrence and/or complete agreement
2 points for frequent occurrence
1 point for occasional occurrence
0 points for no occurrence

Test 1:
Basic Type Classification

		Lung (Wind)	Tripa (Bile)	Péken (Phlegm)
1)	Age:	Over 60 years	15-60 years	Up to 15 years
2)	Height (female)	Over 71 inches	63-71 inches	Up to 63 inches
	(male)	Over 73 inches	67-73 inches	Up to 67 inches
3)	Build:	Slender, fine-boned (may have stooped posture)	Athletic, muscular	Stocky (tendency to be over-weight)
4)	Residential area:	Mountainous/cool, drafty/windy	Hot (dry)	Damp/ sticky
Behavior patterns:				
5)	Sleep:	Light sleep, tends to be sleepless	No sleep problems	Deep sleep, problems with waking up, much sleep

6) Disposition:	Tends to worry and be fearful	Quick to anger, irritable	Tends to be apathetic
7)	Spontaneous	Impatient	Very patient
8) Speech:	Talkative	Heated in conversation	Inattentive
9) Voice:	High, thin	Clear	Pleasant-sounding, deep
10) Skin:	Thin, dry, chapped, rough, cold	Moist, warm, pigment spots	Large-pored, moist, cold, soft
11) Perspiration:	Little tendency, without smell	Strong tendency, intense smell	Average tendency, little smell
12) Activity:	Very active, quick	Motivated, goal-oriented	Certain, slow
13) Fear of:	Wind/cold; likes warmth	Heat/sun	Cold dampness/ likes warmth
14) Sexuality:	Level of desire fluctuates greatly	Passionate, very dominant	Tends to have less desire, but has staying power
15) Hobbies:	Artistic activities, dancing	Competitive sports, hunting	Loafing, reading, taking walks

Overall number of points:

The bodily energy with the highest number of points corresponds to your predominant constitutional energy, which means your basic type. Mixtures of body types in every form are possible. This test just presents a brief profile. Please consult the respective sections of the book, especially the chapters on dietary and behavior patterns, as well as pulse and urine analysis, for additional aspects.

Test 2:
Possible Imbalance of a Bodily Energy

Lung (Wind)	Tripa (Bile)	Péken (Phlegm)
Activities before symptoms occurred, etc.		
1) Was exposed to wind/cold	Was exposed to heat	Was exposed to dampness
2) Much mental work or television/computer	Much physical work or sports	Little work or exercise
Food eaten previously		
3) Light and cool food	Hot food or alcohol	Heavy and oily or fatty food
Area of complaints		
4) Hips	Headaches	Sensation of fullness in abdominal area
5) Lower back/ kidney area	Shooting pain in upper portion of body	Digestive complaints/ flatulence
6) Frequent yawning, stretching, shivering	Bitter taste in mouth	Food has no taste
7) Mental instability/ nervousness/twitching	"Being under pressure"	Sensation of heaviness in body and mind
Preferred tastes		
8) Sweet Sweet Sour Bitter Bitter Astringent Hot Cool	Hot Sour Astringent Coarse	
All symptoms worsen		
9) Morning	Noon	Evening
All symptoms worsen		
10) When hungry	During digestion	1 hour after eating
All symptoms improve when		
11) Food is warm and oily	Food is cool	Food is warm

12) Surroundings are warm and pleasant, calm, enjoyable conversations	Surroundings are cool	Surroundings are warm

Overall number of points:
The bodily energy with the highest number of points indicates an excess and obstructs the other bodily energies as a result. In order to more precisely classify the bodily energies, please read the respective chapters (above all, the chapters on dietary and behavior patterns, as well as pulse and urine analysis) on the additional specifics, symptoms, etc. The possibilities for positive influences are primarily found in the chapter on behavior and dietary patterns (see page 89f.).

Selected Bibliography

Arya, P.Y. (1998): *Dictionary of Tibetan Materia Medica*. New Delhi: Motilal Banarsidass.

Badmajeff, W. (1994): *Lung-Tripa-Bakan*. Ulm: Fabri.

Birnbaum, R., Eaton J., Blofeld C. (1980). *The Healing Buddha*. Boston: Shambala.

Clark, B. (1995): *The Quintessence Tantras of Tibetan Medicine*. Ithaca, New York: Snow Lion Publications.

Clifford, T. (1984): *Tibetan Buddhist Medicine and Psychiatry (The Diamond Healing)*. York Beach, ME: Samuel Weiser.

Cornu, P. (1997): *Tibetan Astrology*. Boston & London: Shambala.

Donden Y. (1986): *Health through Balance*. Ithaca, New York: Snow Lion Publications.

Donden, Y. and Kelsang, J. (1983): *The Ambrosia Heart Tantra*. Dharamsala: Library of Tibetan Works and Archives.

Dummer, T. (1988): *Tibetan Medicine and Other Holistic Health-Care Systems*. New Delhi: Paljor Publications.

Finck, E. (1988): *Studies in Tibetan Medicine*. Ithaca, New York: Snow Lion Publications.

Meyer, F. (Editor) (1992): *Tibetan Medical Paintings. Illustrations to the Blue Beryl Treatise of Sangye Gyamtso (1653-1705)*. London: Harry N. Abrams.

Sogyal Rinpoche (1992): *The Tibetan Book of Living and Dying*. San Francisco: Harper Collins.

Tarthang T. (1978): *Kum Nye Relaxation*. Dharma Publishing.

Thurman, R.F. (translator)(1994): *The Tibetan Book of the Dead*. New York: Bantam Doubleday Dell Publications.

Tibetan Medicine, Series 1-9 (1980-1985). Dharamsala: Library of Tibetan Works and Archives.

Trungpa, C. (1981): Journey without Goal. Boulder & London: Prajna Press.

Tsarong, T.J. (1994): *Tibetan Medicinal Plants*. Kalimpong: Tibetan Medical Publications.

Addresses

Padma Health Products, Inc.
Martin Wolf, Vice President
215 River Vale Road,
River Vale, New Jersey 07675
Phone: (201) 664-2100
Fax: (201) 666-8470
Tollfree: 1-877-877-2362
martinwolf@padma-usa.com
http://www.padma-usa.com
Producers and distributors of Padma Basic and other Padma health products in the USA.

TibetMed
http://www.tibetmed.org
Tibetan medicine website featuring Ask Dr. Namseling, archives of the First International Congress on Tibetan Medicine, Washington, DC, November 1998, and an extensive listing of related links. This site is the gateway to many more resources.

Alternative Medicine Foundation, Inc
5411 West Cedar Lane, Suite 205-A
Bethesda, MD 20814
Tel: 301-581-0116
Fax: 301-581-0119
email: amfi@amfoundation.org
http://amfoundation.org
Information resources on alternative and complementary medicine includes a resource Guide on Tibetan medicine.

Herb Research Foundation
1007 Pearl Street, Suite 200
Boulder, CO 80302
Tel: 303-449-2265
Fax: 303-449-7849
info@herbs.org
http://www.herbs.org
Research resources for herbal supplements including Tibetan herbal supplements.

International Tibetan Medical Association (ITMA)
Wainwright House
260 Stuyvesant Ave.
Rye, NY 10580
General Information: 914-967-6080 ext. 1465
Fax: 914-967-6114
itma@meditma.org
http://www.meditma.org
National association for practitioners, researchers and all who are interested in supporting Tibetan medicine in the USA.

Internatural
(Retail)
33719 116th Street
Twin Lakes, WI 53181 USA
800 643 4221 (toll free order line)
262 889 8581 office phone
WEB SITE: www.internatural.com
Web site includes an extensive annotated catalog of more than 7000 products that can be ordered "on line" for your convenience 24 hours a day, 7 days a week.
Retail source of: *Tibetan*, Ayurvedic and other health related herbs, supplements and personal care products.

Lotus Light Enterprises, Inc.
(Wholesale)
P. O. Box 1008
Silver Lake, WI 531 70 USA
262 889 8501 (phone)
262 889 8591 (fax)
800 548 3824 (toll free order line)
Offers an extensive selection of useful products, including: *Tibetan*, Ayurvedic and other health related herbs, natural body care, aromatherapy, flower essences, crystals and tumbled stones, homeopathy, herbal products, vitamins and supplements, videos, books, audio tapes, candles, incense and bulk herbs, teas, massage tools and products and numerous alternative health items across a wide range of categories.